BONE MARROW TRANSPLANTS

BONE MARROW TRANSPLANTS

······································

A Guide for Cancer Patients and Their Families

Marianne L. Shaffer, R.N.
Foreword by George W. Santos, M.D.

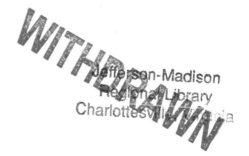

TAYLOR PUBLISHING COMPANY
Dallas, Texas

1361 0017

Published by Taylor Publishing Company
1550 West Mockingbird Lane
Dallas, Texas 75235

Note: some medical terms in this book have been slightly simplified for a general readership.

Library of Congress Cataloging-in-Publication Data

Shaffer, Marianne L.
    Bone marrow transplants : a guide for cancer patients and their families / Marianne L. Shaffer ; foreword by George W. Santos.
        p.   cm.
    Includes bibliographical references and index.
    ISBN 0-87833-855-1   —ISBN 0-87833-854-3 (pbk.)
    1. Bone marrow—Transplantation—Popular works.   I. Title.
    RD123.5.S53—1993
    617.4'4—dc20   93-23704
                                                                          CIP

Printed in the United States of America

10 9 8 7 6 5 4 3 2

To my husband, Tim, for your patience, support, and loyalty. You've always been at my side to give an encouraging smile, a word of praise, or a shoulder to cry on. Your unconditional love gives me the strength to face adversity and someone with whom to share the joy of life's victories. I will always love you.

And to my son, Kevin, for your easy smile, your marvelous sense of humor, and the patience and understanding you show that are beyond your years. You give me the greatest joy a mother can know, that of watching you grow and succeed in life.

Contents

· · · · · · · · · · · · · · · ·

Foreword

· · · · · · · · · · · · · · · · · · ·

The historical roots of bone marrow transplantation can be traced back to the early part of the twentieth century. In 1922 Fabricious-Moeller, a Danish investigator, noted that the platelet depression and bleeding complications following total body irradiation (high-dose radiation therapy administered to the entire body) could be avoided by the simple maneuver of shielding the legs of irradiated guinea pigs. The importance of this early observation was not appreciated and, indeed, forgotten.

Twenty-seven years later, Jacobson and his coworkers made a similar observation in mice exposed to lethal total body irradiation. The platelet and white blood cell depressions, and their ensuing lethal consequences, could be prevented by shielding the spleen (a blood-forming organ in the mouse) from the radiation. It was subsequently shown that cells in the shielded spleen or leg bones migrated to repopulate the bone marrow of the irradiated animals. It was soon discovered that marrow from normal animals could be harvested and transfused intravenously into lethally irradiated animals—with life-saving results.

From the late fifties to the late sixties, bone marrow transplantation was performed in patients in the end stages of their disease. They most often were experiencing a full relapse of their disease, and many had accompanying infections. Despite a failure rate of 85% to 90%, 10% to 15% of the leukemic patients were cured. In the early seventies, patients underwent transplants while in remission and the results improved markedly.

Although total body irradiation had been the major method employed to prepare patients for transplantation, we at Johns Hopkins and other researchers developed alternative regimens, some of which (such as busulfan and cyclophosphamide) did not require total body irradiation.

In the eighties, the clinical outcomes continued to improve with better prevention and control of severe graft-versus-host disease (GVHD). The establishment of the National Marrow Donor Program for unrelated donors and the development of autologous (self) bone marrow transplantation for the lymphomas, acute leukemias, and other diseases allowed more patients to be considered for transplantation. With the improvements in supportive care, better ways to prevent and manage GVHD, and the use of autologous transplantation, older patients could be offered the procedure as well.

The development of bone marrow transplantation for the treatment of human disease has been an exciting adventure for many of us. I am particularly gratified to be able to write this foreword for Marianne Shaffer, a previous patient of mine. As a nurse and former bone marrow transplant patient, she is uniquely qualified to write this volume.

This book is very inclusive and covers the initial emotional response a patient experiences when given the diagnosis of cancer to the organic and psychological long-term effects of the transplantation. Throughout the book, she speaks with the authority and insight of personal experience as well as one who has researched her subject well indeed. She has included helpful suggestions for coping with many of the problems involved with transplantations. This comprehensive guide can serve as an excellent reference for those caring for and those undergoing bone marrow transplantation.

GEORGE W. SANTOS, M.D.
Professor of Oncology and Medicine
Director of Bone Marrow Transplantation Program
JOHNS HOPKINS ONCOLOGY CENTER

Acknowledgments

This book would not have been possible without the assistance and support of so many special people.

First and foremost, I would like to thank my sister, Christine Metcalfe, for the devoted interest and care she showed in support of this project. I am deeply grateful for the countless hours she spent reading, editing, and brainstorming with me to clarify the rough draft, all accomplished in spite of her extraordinarily busy personal and professional life.

I am especially thankful to Natasha Kern, my literary agent, who saw the merit of bringing information on this topic to the public and introduced me to a fantastic editor at Taylor Publishing Company, Lorena Jones, who has not only been a delight to work with, but has shown tireless enthusiasm and support for this project from start to finish.

My sincere thanks to Dr. George W. Santos for writing the book's foreword and for taking the time to read through the manuscript to help ensure its medical accuracy. I am profoundly grateful for the dedicated work he and others have given to the field of bone marrow transplantation to make this procedure successful for individuals like myself.

A loving thanks to my parents, John and Nancy Martin, and to my husband, Tim, for their contributions to this book through their valuable comments, suggestions, patience, and support; and a special thank-you to my sister, Susan DiPaula, for writing the "Donor's Message" found in chapter 2.

I also wish to thank the following individuals, who supported and cared for me throughout my illness and recovery, without whom the opportunity to share what I have learned with others ultimately would not have been possible:

Dr. Georgia B. Vogelsang; Dr. Richard J. Jones; Dr. Greg Kalemkarian; Dawn Miller, PA-C; Suzanne Demko, PA-C; Joy L. Fincannon, R.N.; Laura Deforge, R.N.; Lori Summerson, R.N.; Viki Altomonte, R.N.; Joanne Wohlganger, R.N.; Terry Moorman, R.N.; Trisha Sigley, R.D., L.D.; Stacy Czerwinski, P.T.; Adrienne Polland; and all of the other skilled, caring professionals at the . Johns Hopkins Oncology Center who participated in my care.

Dr. A. Thomas Andrews, Dr. Shashikant B. Patel, Dr. Kathryn Peroutka, and their outstanding oncology nurses and office staff.

Dr. John D. Conroy, Jr., for his excellent pretransplant and post-BMT medical care.

Dr. David R. Halbert; Dr. Gerald Woodward; Dr. Robert J. Kantor; Dr. Manuel F. Quesada; Dr. Sherna D. Bharucha; Marie Christie, B.S.W.; Sandy O'Sullivan, R.N.; Pat Kile, R.N.; Robin Martinez; Brenda Smith, R.N.; the nurses of the I.V. Team; Carol Rowan, R.N.; Linda Books, L.P.N.; Charlotte Rabuck, L.P.N.; and all of the other nurses, staff members, and former colleagues of mine at the Harrisburg Hospital for their excellent care and words of encouragement.

Dr. Howard R. Cohen and his caring nurses and office staff.

Pastor J. Gerald Greiner and my "church family" at the Mechanicsburg Church of the Brethren for their devoted support, cards, and prayers.

Rosemary Schaedler, Nancy Karlik Surridge, and all of my friends at the American Cancer Society's PA Division office, Cumberland Unit, and CanSurmount Support Group.

Nancy Roth, my "BMT buddy," for listening and understanding as few others can.

Fran Coffman; Dorothy Dailey, R.N.; J. Robert Johnston; James H. Metcalfe; Brian Weller; Steven L.T. DiPaula; David and Linda Borch; my in-laws, Hope and Elmer Shaffer, and the entire Shaffer family; the Mechanicsburg Education Association; the staff of the Mechanicsburg Learning Center; Denise and Robert Ward; Lynn Michels, R.N.; Lisa Leen, R.T.R.M.; my many platelet and blood donor volunteers; and all of my other friends, and those of my family, who supported us in our time of need. You are too numerous to name, but will never be forgotten for your caring and generosity.

Finally, my heartfelt thanks to Christine for mothering Kevin when I was unable and for the indispensable help and care that she gave so freely to me and my family; to Susan for donating the marrow that gave me a second chance at life—we will always share a special bond; to Tim and Kevin, whose steadfast love and devotion always gave me the will to keep fighting toward recovery; and to my parents for their unwavering help and support, innumerable sacrifices made on my behalf, lifelong encouragement that taught me to believe in myself, and strong foundation of love that showed me how to face adversity with courage, grace, and hope.

Introduction

· ·

In the spring of 1989, I was much like other women I knew who were around my age. I was happily married, with a 3-year-old son and another child on the way. But that year, the first week of June heralded in a series of events that irrevocably changed my life. At 32 years of age, I was diagnosed with acute myelomonocytic leukemia. My cancer was discovered "accidentally" after what should have been a happy event in our lives. Nine weeks into my pregnancy, my husband and I went to the office of my obstetrician to hear the heartbeat of our growing child, the child it had taken us 6 months to conceive.

After an unsuccessful attempt by my doctor to find the baby's heartbeat, he suggested that I have a sonogram just to be sure nothing was wrong. My appointment was scheduled within the hour at a nearby testing facility. After a little searching, the technician found the image of our baby. She continued to scan and get different views, but neither of us mentioned for a few minutes what the lack of movement meant. Then she gently told us that there was no heartbeat, but that the size indicated the baby had died just within the past few days. A phone call was placed to my obstetrician, who expressed his condolences and scheduled a therapeutic abortion at the local hospital where I had once worked.

My husband and I were devastated. We could hardly believe this had happened to us. It seemed these things always happened to someone else. We had taken for granted our happy, comfortable life. As difficult as it was, we did our best to explain the loss of the baby to our young son. I'll never forget how he tried to comfort me by saying we could "get a new, better baby." Thinking that this was the worst that could happen to us, we went home and mourned our loss. Little did we know, or even fathom, that this event would soon be overshadowed by another life-altering tragedy which awaited us around the next bend.

Two days later at the hospital, as I was wheeled into the Operating Room, my obstetrician told me that my bloodwork showed that my red blood cell count was low. He said it should not be this low so early in my pregnancy. He recommended that I call a hematologist when I got home for an evaluation to examine the cause. I told him that I had been very tired for many months with a persistent winter cold that I just couldn't seem to shake. I also had an enlarged lymph node on one side of my neck, shortness of breath with activity, and various aches and pains in my chest and back. I suppose I should have realized something was seriously wrong, particularly since I am a nurse, but my symptoms were just so vague and flulike. Several weeks before, I had gone to my family doctor, but he too figured I just had a lingering upper respiratory infection.

Although I was concerned to discover that my red blood cell count was so low, I still figured it must have something to do with the pregnancy that had gone awry. After I returned from the Operating Room, I started to feel extremely chilled and spiked a temperature of around 104°. My anesthesiologist was notified, and she ordered a chest X ray and bloodwork, including a complete blood count (CBC). It was then she told me that I had experienced some problems while under the anesthesia. She had needed to frequently suction my airway because I had copious amounts of respiratory secretions. In addition, I had a number of spasms of my larynx, which caused me to temporarily stop breathing.

I was frightened and surmised that I must have bronchitis, pneumonia, or some other type of respiratory infection. Little did I realize at the time that my problem was far more serious than that. It didn't take long, however, to find out what was wrong. Soon after my bloodwork was done, a procession of medical personnel entered my room and surrounded my bed. I started to feel scared. It didn't take three doctors and a few nurses to tell me I had pneumonia.

The medical internist spoke first and quoted all of my labwork, assuming perhaps that I'd know what a low red blood cell count and a twice normal white blood cell count with numerous blast cells meant. I asked him just what he thought was wrong, and he answered that it looked like I had acute granulocytic leukemia. After being seen by an oncologist and undergoing a bone marrow aspiration and biopsy, it was indeed confirmed that I had a type of acute leukemia. All in one week, I lost my baby and had to face the possibility of losing my own life as well. I was in a state of shock at how quickly my seemingly secure life had changed.

I remained in the hospital for the next 2 months. I was plunged into a world of chemotherapy, protective isolation, illness, and fear. Before a remission from the disease was even attained, my doctors began to talk to me about the potential benefits of undergoing a bone marrow transplant (BMT). Oncology was not my field, and I couldn't even remember from nursing school what a bone marrow transplant was. After the procedure was explained, my parents spoke up and said that they already knew my older sister, Susan, was a "perfect" donor match. This had been determined from confidential testing that was done a decade before.

Susan had been afflicted with kidney disease late in childhood. Because my younger sister, Christine, and I were relatively young when Sue's kidneys eventually failed, my parents decided to have the doctors try a transplant using an unrelated kidney donor instead of having another child undergo major surgery. After two attempts, she had a successful kidney transplant. In retrospect, my physicians were glad my parents had made that decision so many years ago. This way I still had both of my kidneys to face the barrage of intensive treatment that lay ahead.

After undergoing two rounds of chemotherapy to get into remission and one round of consolidation chemotherapy to maintain it, I was evaluated and accepted for bone marrow transplant treatment at the Johns Hopkins Oncology Center in Baltimore, Maryland, in the fall of 1989. It was there that I met Dr. George W. Santos, a deeply compassionate man who has dedicated his life to saving the lives of people like me through his miraculous work in the field of hematology and bone marrow transplantation. My transplant took place on October 10, 1989. With a combination of excellent medical care, loving family and friends, the good Lord above, and a large dose of luck, I survived and am leukemia-free today.

Since the first successful bone marrow transplant in 1968, bone marrow transplantation has been evolving into a treatment that today offers the hope of a cure to thousands. Most would have had little or no chance of surviving if diagnosed just a few decades ago. Unfortunately, only about 30% of the patients who could potentially benefit from a transplant using donor marrow have a related donor match. The odds of finding a donor match among the general population are only about 1 in 20,000 and can be up to 1 in a million depending upon the patient's genetic background. That's why organizations like the National Marrow Donor Program and others have worked so valiantly to encourage more people to have their names added to a registry of potential marrow donors. BMT can be the only hope some patients with life-threatening illnesses have in getting a second chance at life.

Although I felt rather alone when first diagnosed with leukemia, I have learned since then that I had just joined the ranks of more than 29,000 cases of leukemia and 1 million cases of cancer that are diagnosed each year in this country. According to present rates, about 1 in 3 Americans (approximately 85 million Americans) will eventually have cancer.* Because the vast majority of bone marrow transplants are done to treat cancer, I have chosen to devote this book to that group of diseases. Those who are treated for other diseases will still find much of the information relevant, however, because of the many similarities found in BMT treatments.

This book is in no way intended to take the place of a physician or to recommend BMT as a treatment for you. Only your physician, together with you and your family, can make that decision. If you

---

*Statistics taken from the American Cancer Society's *Cancer Facts & Figures—1993.*

have had a BMT or are considering one, it is important that you follow the specific instructions and recommendations given to you by your physician and BMT center. Not all of the information contained in this book will be applicable to your situation. Check with your physician if you have questions. Consider also that in an evolving field such as this, you are bound to find changes both within and among BMT centers as research continues.

Even though there has been an increase in the information presented to the public about bone marrow transplantation through stories featured in newspapers, magazines, television shows, and movies, there are still many misconceptions about this procedure. Many people think that it involves cutting open the bones to remove or insert marrow. They don't know that the marrow is transplanted into the recipient through an intravenous (I.V.) line, much like a bag of blood is given. Because so many people have asked me questions about this procedure since my own transplant and expressed the same frustration I have at the lack of published information available in local libraries and bookstores about BMT, I felt compelled to share what I have learned through my own experience and research.

There is a great deal of information contained in this book. Even with the best of explanations, some aspects about bone marrow transplantation are exceedingly complex, so take your time and read at your own pace. Learn as much or as little as you want. If you choose, just read the information that pertains to your present situation, and save the rest for later. If you find it upsetting to read about side effects or potential complications, then skip over or just skim those sections. I know just how difficult and overwhelming learning about BMT, undergoing the treatment, and recovering from the procedure can be. I hope this book will provide you with the information you are seeking and will lead you to other resources and organizations that will prove helpful in easing your journey through the BMT experience.

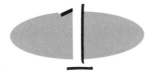

When the Diagnosis Is Cancer

· · · · · · · · · · · · · · ·

CANCER. What kind of thoughts pass through your mind when you hear this word? Because a diagnosis of cancer often evokes fearful images of suffering, pain, and death, it is important to first address some of the feelings that can accompany being told you have cancer and to emphasize the fact that many people, like myself, have been cured of cancer and have gone on to resume healthy, productive lives.

Examining your feelings, creating an atmosphere of openness with your loved ones, learning about your disease, and coming to terms with the fact that you have cancer can greatly aid you and your family in facing the difficult times that lie ahead. These are not, however, easy things for most of us to do. I hope the information I share with you throughout this chapter will help you discover additional ways of coping with cancer and its treatment and provide you with some new sources to utilize to increase your knowledge.

The Emotional Response

Almost all of us have known others who have had cancer. Their experiences often color our own emotional response to cancer. I know, before my illness, I incorrectly equated the diagnosis of cancer with almost certain death. I did not work in the field of oncology, and the cancer patients that I did happen to see when I worked at a local hospital were usually either undergoing intensive treatments or were dying. I did not see those who regained their health and knew few cancer survivors myself. The information in my medical textbooks from nursing school was written over a decade before my own diagnosis and did not reflect new advances and treatment options. I was not fully aware of all of the progress that has been made in combating many of the different types of cancer.

This emphasizes how important it is to have current information and to avoid letting the negative experiences of some cancer patients rob you of hope for your own recovery, particularly if these experiences were a long time ago. Hope is an essential element in the battle against cancer. It keeps you from sinking into despair and gives you the will to fight. It does not mean that you are denying the reality of your illness, just that you are striving toward a future where you are once again well.

Soon after my diagnosis, one of my physicians arranged for a former leukemia patient to come into the hospital to talk to me. He had been diagnosed 5 years before and was now considered cured. Meeting and talking to others who have been through what you face can help you feel more hopeful about your chances for recovery. It may also ease some of the fear and isolation that a diagnosis of cancer can cause. If you believe this would benefit you, ask your physician if he or she knows a patient who would talk with you. If not, check with your local chapter of the American Cancer Society or with other cancer organizations in your area that offer support services.

Even with a great deal of support and encouragement, facing the fact that you have a life-threatening illness is not easy. It can be additionally difficult if bone marrow transplantation (BMT) is recommended because your cancer has not or does not respond well to conventional treatments. BMT is not only an extremely physically demanding treatment but is an especially psychologically demanding one as well. It may be even more difficult if it follows closely on the heels of your initial diagnosis, as it often does for those with certain acute types of cancer.

Shock and denial are common initial reactions to finding out you have cancer. A life change as drastic as this requires time to adjust to, for it rocks the secure foundation of your day-to-day life. It's normal to cry and feel sad. We all need time to grieve over the loss of our health and the loss of our "innocence" about our mortality. Even though we all know that we will die someday, facing the fact that it could be sooner, rather than later, is quite a jolt.

I'll never forget how I felt when I was told that I had leukemia. My first reaction was that there had to be some mistake. My test results were probably mixed up with someone else's. I even asked if this could be confused with some other diagnosis. I just couldn't believe that something like this could happen to me.

On one of the days soon after I was told of my disease, a social worker brought me a number of books that listed resource agencies for cancer patients. At first, I couldn't fathom why I would need books targeted toward cancer patients. I had *leukemia,* not *cancer!* I was told and knew that leukemia is a cancer of the blood-forming tissues, yet, emotionally, I just wasn't ready to face it. Leukemia seemed like a separate blood disease that had nothing to do with cancer. After all, the name cancer wasn't anywhere in the name of the disease as it is in some other kinds of cancer, like breast cancer or prostate cancer.

I know now that the initial denial I felt was just one of the ways my brain was protecting me from more than I was able to handle at the time. Don't be too hard on yourself if you've experienced similar feelings. They are quite normal. Give yourself time to adjust. It is often hard to talk about your feelings or to even know exactly what you are feeling in the beginning. This confusion may be increased by the massive quantity of new information you are bombarded with during this period. Emotional turmoil makes it even more difficult to concentrate and absorb all of the details that accompany explanations about your illness. Time usually aids most people in assimilating this information, however, and in accepting, or beginning to accept, the reality of their diagnosis.

When you feel ready, take an active role by asking questions and learning more about your disease and its treatment. Knowledge can be a powerful tool in that it teaches you ways to help yourself. If the stress of your situation gets too overwhelming, learn relaxation techniques you can use to help defuse it. Listening to uplifting tapes and reading books that focus on the positive are helpful for some people. Keeping journals or writing poetry to express feelings are useful to others.

I found that talking openly about my cancer and hearing loved ones discuss what they were feeling helped give me the support I needed to better accept and cope with what was happening in my life. I relied heavily on the many good listeners I was fortunate to know who helped me sort through the barrage of feelings that were swirling around inside of me.

Although cancer is not the taboo word today it was decades ago, fear of the word can still trigger an immediate response that makes it difficult for some patients and families to talk about it openly. A first reaction in some families is to try and protect one another by not discussing it. This is why families sometimes don't want Mother, Dad, or the children to know. These secrets can lead to resentment and a lack of trust later on. Try to put yourself in the place of another family member and imagine how you would feel if secrets about a loved one's health were kept from you.

Regardless of how strong you are emotionally, fear and even terror or panic are normal reactions when your life is threatened. Fear may particularly surface as protective mechanisms of disbelief and denial fade. Confronting your fears and talking about them can help keep them from escalating and immobilizing you. I tried to combat my own fear by thinking of things I could do to keep my mind occupied. Find activities and distractions that work for you. This is particularly useful at bedtime, when stress and fear can cause insomnia. Develop a relaxation routine that helps clear your mind and push away worry.

Although I tried to remain positive and strong to fight my cancer, there were times when I became too physically or emotionally exhausted to keep from temporarily sinking into depression. It is normal to feel this way, particularly when so many things in your life seem out of control. I found that most days were like an emotional roller coaster filled with ups and downs. It is important to realize that some medications you may be receiving as part of your treatment can contribute to emotional instability as well. The temporary havoc some drugs can wreak on your mental status can be very scary, especially if you are unaware in advance that this may occur.

I found that participating in my own care, and making as many decisions as I could, helped push away some of the depression. It helped me feel more in control of my life. Taking an assertive approach to coping with your illness can help keep you from feeling sorry for yourself. A positive attitude and a strong will to live are essential weapons in the fight against cancer.

Maintaining as normal a lifestyle as possible can also keep you from obsessively focusing on your illness. The kind of cancer you have, though, often determines whether this is a realistic goal. It depends on the type of treatment you have: Whether it is inpatient or outpatient treatment; if it involves surgery, radiation therapy, and/or chemotherapy; and the severity of the side effects. Some cancer patients are able to continue working, maintaining a home, caring for children, etc., while undergoing treatments.

The part of your body affected by the cancer and its treatment, as well as the accompanying changes in body image, affect how you cope with your illness, too. Many patients experience hair loss as a result of their anticancer therapy. Physique changes range from excessive thinness to bloating and weight gain. Surgery results in incisional lines and sometimes brings about dramatic body changes. Adjusting to these alterations in your "normal" appearance can be temporarily demoralizing. Furthermore, becoming debilitated and having to rely on others for your care can heighten feelings of abnormality and dependency. Your stage of life, level of maturity, and self-esteem prior to becoming ill are all important factors that can influence how well you cope with the physical and emotional ramifications of having cancer.

Even in the most rational and mature of persons, however, feelings of anger, guilt, and jealousy are not uncommon. During my own illness, at times I felt envious of people who were happy and healthy, and angry if they seemed not to appreciate how lucky they were. I also felt a tremendous sense of injustice. I was in the prime of my life with unfulfilled goals and a child to raise. My life was now irrevocably changed, and I felt angry that this had happened.

If you find yourself getting angry at others, try to deduce whether you are truly angry at some event that occurred, or if you're just venting feelings that are bottled up inside. Apologizing, if you have treated someone unfairly, can go a long way in reestablishing communication at a time when it is so essential. Being ill does not give one license to treat loved ones or others unkindly, even though we might feel angry with them or the rest of the "healthy" world for not having to go through what we are experiencing.

Then again, patients who are under the influences of potent drugs and extreme stress should not be held accountable if their behavior is not what is normally considered socially acceptable. Family members and friends need to understand this, so they won't be offended or harbor anger or grudges against a patient for things the patient may not even remember saying or doing during his or her treatment. As soon as possible, both patient and family members need to talk with one another and resolve any issues that are bothering them so their relationships are not negatively affected months or years later.

In spite of the fact that it was not my fault that I got leukemia, at times I felt guilty about what I was putting my family through (although this only served to make me feel worse than I already did). Try not to place blame on others or blame yourself for becoming ill, even if you come across some "inspirational" books that attribute your state of mind at the time as a contributing factor in your developing cancer. This unnecessary guilt only serves to increase what is already a tremendous emotional burden to bear. Even if a particular lifestyle or behavior may have contributed to the cancer, such as being diagnosed with lung cancer after years of smoking, guilt and blame are best put aside because they are only destructive after the fact and help neither the patient nor family in the long run.

Finally, determination to fight for a cure does not preclude confronting and talking about the possibility of dying. Sometimes these thoughts are kept hidden from loved ones because you don't want to upset them. If this is important for you to discuss, let your family know that it's okay to talk about this with you, or if necessary, find others with whom to discuss these concerns. Before I was admitted for my transplant, my husband and I talked about some of the things

I would want, such as who would help care for our son, in case things did not go as we hoped.

Not all patients or families can or want to discuss things such as these. I'm not suggesting you should if you feel no need to do so, or view it as too detrimental to your morale. I only know that it helped me to get these thoughts and feelings out in the open, instead of leaving them unsaid. The importance of maintaining open communication on all of the issues that accompany life-threatening illness, no matter how painful, proved to be valuable to me.

Although I've just scratched the surface of some of the feelings cancer patients experience, I believe it is an appropriate place to start when discussing the subject of bone marrow transplantation. Having a transplant places inordinate stresses on both patient and family alike. Even with a great deal of emotional strength and open communication, it is a tough treatment regimen to get through. It is important to examine where you and your family are in regard to your coping skills, how open you are when talking with one another, and if you need counseling or support services before beginning the transplant experience. What truly helped me cope in my battle against leukemia was a loving family, caring friends, and supportive medical professionals. The role and importance of a good support system cannot be overemphasized.

Evaluating Support Systems

A person's support system comes into play from the very moment a diagnosis of cancer is made. If a person is alone at the time, who does he or she tell first? If a person is with someone else at the time, who is it? Human beings are naturally social beings who rejoice with one another when happy and turn to one another for support and comfort in times of tragedy, sorrow, and grief. Relationships with others are often complex, each accompanied by a unique history all their own. I can think of no greater test that validates or invalidates the strength of these relationships than being plunged into intense adversity, such as that which life-threatening illness brings.

The Family

My family and I were told by a social worker soon after arriving at Johns Hopkins that the treatment regimen and lengthy recovery time associated with a bone marrow transplant most often drew families closer together or became the final straw that tore them apart. Examining how functional a family is before facing a crisis such as this is a good place to start in predicting how the members will react when confronted with the extreme stresses inherent in bone marrow transplantation.

Most people turn to members of their family first for the support they need. I was lucky enough to have a loving, supportive husband, two marvelous parents who unselfishly gave their time and energies, and two siblings who love me deeply. They participated in my care and my son's care and supported each other throughout this ordeal.

That's not to say that it was easy or that great sacrifices weren't made. Even in the best of families, bickering and resentments can surface as stress mounts. Family members can become critical of the way one person does something or angry at an apparent imbalance in the work load. Nitpicking and gossiping among family members about another only serves to tear away at the teamwork that is so essential at this time. It can be quite difficult to overlook these negative feelings as inequities and friction arise. Nevertheless, try to recognize the contributions each family member can make or is willing to make, instead of focusing on what he or she cannot or chooses not to do.

Each person is a unique individual with his or her own strengths and weaknesses. No one person can or should be expected to do it all. Whereas one family member may be excellent at providing child care, another may not have the patience or desire to participate in this way at all. One family member may have great job flexibility and be able to take time off; another may severely jeopardize his or her livelihood by attempting to take off the same amount of time. Geographical limitations must also be taken into consideration.

It is important for a family to discuss these issues as plans are being made for the transplant. Holding a family meeting for all the parties involved can serve to lay the groundwork for not only reviewing tasks and needs of the patient and family but for establishing and renewing an open dialogue amongst members that can hopefully be maintained throughout the following months.

When added pressure and responsibility go on for an extended period of time, family members often become physically and emotionally exhausted. They can develop all kinds of distressing symptoms from the unrelenting demands that are placed upon them. For example, my husband developed neck and back pain that became so severe he was forced to see a physician for treatment. Although so much of the focus is naturally on the patient's illness at a time like this, family members must recognize signs that tell them to slow down or seek help for physical or emotional problems.

To come through this experience with a strong, intact family unit requires open, effective communication which is, ideally, intertwined with love, respect, understanding, and forgiveness for each other. Unfortunately, not everyone is as blessed as I was with this kind of family support and must look elsewhere in their time of need.

Friends

A logical second place to look for support is to turn to friends, particularly if you do not have family living nearby or who are willing to help. There are some family members who might make an initial show of support, but when the going gets rough they get going and disappear as well. The same can be true for friends. You will soon learn who your true friends are. Your network of acquaintances and friends need not be extensive, because it is the quality of these friendships, not the quantity, that is important. Some cancer patients, however, talk of losing friends after their diagnosis. Sometimes a relationship just does not survive if it delves too far below the superficial or pleasant aspects of life. These relationships are usually the first to be severed when cancer enters your life.

Occasionally, someone that you thought was a good friend will move to the fringes of your life. Quite possibly, it is not because they don't truly care about you, but because they feel too unsure about what to say or do. Sometimes your diagnosis can make them feel extremely uncomfortable, because it serves as a vivid reminder of their own mortality. Depending on the person, it may be too difficult for him or her to talk about the subject of serious illness with you. Friends might also feel guilty when talking to you, particularly if they are quite blessed with health and happiness in their own lives. Just thinking about what would have happened in their own lives if this had happened to them and not to you can be quite overwhelming. They might be reluctant to share what is going on in their lives for fear it may seem trivial compared with the concerns you face. It is also very painful to see someone that you care about suffering, and friends may be grieving over this illness that threatens your life.

There are several ways you can help facilitate communication with friends at this time. If you choose, tell them simply and honestly what has occurred in your life. Don't overwhelm them with details if they don't ask for them. Respect the fact that they might need some time to pull themselves together before seeing you; this can be quite a shock to them as well. Acknowledge their feelings and show understanding, particularly if they admit to not knowing what to say or do.

Don't thrust your needs on them, but when genuine offers of help are made, give concrete ways they can help out, such as dropping off a meal, picking up a child at school, doing a load of laundry, etc. Try not to minimize concerns they might share about things that are going on in their own lives, and try not to take advantage of their kindness. Many people are already overextended and struggling to stay caught up with the pace of modern-day life.

Treat both family and friends with respect, but remember that if a greater burden is placed on friends than they are willing to accept, they may be more likely to walk away from the relationship and not feel the responsibility toward you that a family member does. Remember to tell both family and friends how much you appreciate what they are doing for you and how much it means to you to have them in your life. You may end up being pleasantly surprised at the number of people who step forward with offers of help and support.

Religious and Social Organizations

In times of adversity many people turn to their church or synagogue. If you are already active in a church or synagogue in your community, chances are they will rally behind you and your family at this time of need. Many churches and synagogues have communication networks in place that pass the word about those who are experiencing illness or misfortune to others in the congregation. Most pastors, priests, and rabbis regularly make visits to church members who are hospitalized and offer spiritual support to both patients and families. Depending on your relationship with your religious leader, he or she can be an invaluable listener and a source of great comfort.

Those who do not presently attend church or temple may feel the need to establish or renew religious ties. Life-threatening illness tends to elicit a priority restructuring in most people's lives and religious concerns may be moved to the forefront. Renewed involvement with the church or temple may also be coupled with the need to reconcile troubled relationships with others.

Some people belong to social organizations or clubs that may volunteer help through monetary donations from fund raisers or with offers to help meet a family's needs. Sometimes these contacts provide great support and are really more a part of a patient's network of good friends. For very private people who do not want others in the community to know of their illness, these are not possible sources of support. (No one should contact any group or organization without a patient's approval to do so.)

Human and Social Service Organizations

There are several cancer-related organizations that offer much in the way of educational information. There are even some organizations that provide specific information about BMT. Some of these organizations provide emotional and support services as well, such as support groups, individual support, counseling, legal referrals, or financial aid programs.

Some patients find support groups to be worthwhile in furnishing helpful information, bolstering self-esteem, and providing a place of acceptance and safety to discuss innermost feelings. Encouragement from people who have already been through treatment for cancer can be invaluable in helping you face what lies ahead. Seeing others who have been cured from cancer or who are coping with treatments can help boost your morale and offer hope. Although we all react somewhat differently, most patients find that they share many of the same emotional and physical concerns as others who are battling cancer.

I became active in a local support group soon after my discharge from the hospital and have remained active to this day due to the way it has enriched my life. Support group members can grow to become good and trusted friends. After all, friendships often grow out of shared experiences, and people usually get to know one another quickly in a setting such as this where deep feelings and thoughts are more apt to be discussed.

So where can groups such as this be found? Cancer support groups may be hospital or community based. They may be run by trained professionals or function more as self-help groups. Places to begin your search for such a group are your local unit of the American Cancer Society or other cancer-related organizations. You can also check your local newspaper, where support groups are often listed in the community services section. Call local hospitals and ask if they run cancer support programs. Larger oncology centers and institutions, where bone marrow transplants are done, often have programs as well. Another source to contact when searching for a support group is your oncologist's office. They will usually know of support groups in your area and be able to refer you to the proper person or place to find out more information.

Psychologists and Psychiatrists

If you or your physician feel you need help beyond the emotional support obtained from those around you, or if you are having a great deal of difficulty coping with the changes brought about by your illness, professional support may be needed. Psychologists are counselors trained to help people having problems adjusting to some aspect in their lives. They can provide guidance in problem solving and teach techniques that are useful in stress reduction, such as relaxation exercises or guided imagery. They usually hold a master's degree and can be licensed just like other health care professionals.

A psychiatrist, on the other hand, is a physician who has undergone specialized training in the diagnosis and treatment of mental disorders and diseases. Since psychiatrists are medical doctors, they can prescribe medications, such as antidepressants and antianxiety agents, whereas psychologists cannot.

These professionals may work for hospitals, community mental health centers, social service organizations, home health care agencies, or have a private practice.

Perhaps others in your family will feel the need to seek help from these sources as well. Some families choose individual counseling, and others choose group counseling. Since these services can be very expensive, it is wise to find out if your health insurance covers such treatment before it is initiated so that you know what your costs will be up front.

Gathering the Facts

Soon after I was diagnosed with leukemia, I felt compelled to learn as much as I could about this disease and its treatment. Becoming educated about what was wrong with my body, and learning what could be done to treat and possibly cure it, helped me feel a little more empowered and in control of my life. Gathering knowledge can not only help lessen feelings of dependency by giving you a tangible, active role to play in your illness; it can also help you make more informed decisions about your care.

So where can you find information about cancer and its treatment? The best source is usually an oncologist, a physician who specializes in treating cancer patients. Chances are if your personal family physician was involved in your initial diagnosis, he or she then referred you to an oncologist. Oncologists receive many years of intensive training in the diagnosis and treatment of cancer and can tap into the latest research and clinical trials to provide up-to-date information and care for their patients.

Depending on the patient's age, this physician might be a pediatric oncologist who specializes in treating cancer in children. Other members of the health care team, such as surgeons, radiologists, infection control specialists, nurses, dieticians, and social workers, can also be valuable resources for information about cancer, its treatment, or the supportive care that accompanies it.

In addition to medical professionals, a number of organizations supply information about cancer and its treatment (including the use of bone marrow transplantation). Some provide information about all kinds of cancer, while others specialize in providing information and support to patients having one particular kind of cancer or treatment.

For information on a wide variety of cancers, an obvious source is the American Cancer Society (ACS), which has a network of offices nationwide. Your state and local chapter locations can be found by calling their national toll-free number or by looking in your local phone book. They have numerous pamphlets and teaching materials available, as well as a computerized information system that can be accessed by volunteers to answer your questions. In addition, they sponsor rehabilitation programs specific to breast cancer, laryngectomies, and ostomies, as well as other programs of support for cancer patients, such as CanSurmount. This program provides one-to-one emotional support by pairing cancer patients with specially trained volunteers who are often former cancer patients themselves. In some areas, there are also CanSurmount self-help groups.

The National Cancer Institute (NCI) is another extremely valuable source for information. It is an agency of the Federal Department of U.S. Health and Human Services. A wealth of information and free publications can be obtained by calling their toll-free Cancer Information Service. Some of the materials they publish are booklets in the form of research reports, including an excellent one entitled *Bone Marrow Transplantation*. You can also receive, upon request, an inspirational and informative book entitled *Fighting Cancer* by Annette and Richard Bloch (R.A. Bloch Cancer Foundation, 1985), which many cancer patients find helpful. In addition, the NCI offers a professional service called the Physician Data Query (PDQ). This computerized database system provides doctors with current clinical trial programs and up-to-date information about cancer treatment. Patients can obtain information about clinical trials themselves by calling the Cancer Information Service.

The Leukemia Society of America (LSA) is a national, voluntary organization that provides information on leukemia, lymphoma, and multiple myeloma. They have programs that target education, financial aid, and research. In addition, they sponsor a network of family support groups nationwide, which at last count consisted of 43 groups. There are many informative educational booklets, pamphlets, and other learning aids available from the Leukemia Society. They also publish two free newsletters, *Newsline* (published quarterly) and *society news* (published bimonthly), which contain medical update sections detailing the latest in research and treatment. As you would expect, the Leukemia Society also has literature available on bone marrow transplantation. Contact your local unit to get a copy of their 52-page education booklet entitled *Bone Marrow Transplantation (BMT)*, as well as their two educational videos on this topic. (One video is for adults and one is for children.)

Two relatively new organizations (which were not in existence at the time of my diagnosis) have been established specifically to provide in-depth information and help to bone marrow transplant patients. One is the *BMT Newsletter,* a nonprofit organization that publishes a bimonthly newsletter. The *BMT Newsletter* is written and published by Susan Stewart, a former BMT patient. Each issue focuses on a specific topic related to bone marrow transplantation. There is no charge for patients to have their names added to this newsletter's mailing list.

Another publication available from this author is a 157-page book entitled *Bone Marrow Transplants: A Book of Basics for Patients.* It is an excellent source for detailed yet easily understandable information on BMT that will be mailed to you for a nominal fee. The information in the book and each newsletter has been written with the help of medical advisors across the country and includes contributions from patients who have undergone BMTs. The *BMT Newsletter* also provides information and referrals on issues related to bone marrow transplantation, such as legal referrals (for patients having difficulty with insurance reimbursement) and patient referrals (to link prospective patients with those who have already undergone BMT).

The other new organization designed to address the needs of BMT patients is the National Bone Marrow Transplant Link. Their stated mission is "to reduce the burdens of those affected by bone marrow transplantation and to promote public understanding." This nonprofit, human service organization assists not only patients and their families, but supports continued research and public education, serves as a clearinghouse and resource center for current information on BMT, and advocates insurance coverage for the procedure. This organization also puts prospective BMT patients in need of support and encouragement in touch with others who have already undergone BMT. There's also an organization called the BMT Family Support Network, which will help link patients and family members with others who've been through the experience (see the appendix for more information).

In addition to those just mentioned, there are some other organizations associated with bone marrow transplantation. They focus on transplants that use donors. The National Marrow Donor Program (NMDP), which is a network of more than 100 donor centers throughout the country, was officially established by an Act of Congress in 1987. It was created because many patients in need of a transplant do not have a related donor with a suitable match. This network not only includes donor centers, but transplant centers, collection centers, and recruitment groups. The NMDP currently has over 1 million donor volunteers on file and works with almost 40 countries worldwide.

NMDP is involved in dispensing information about BMT, recruiting donors, performing tissue-typing tests, providing donor counseling and education and studying the effectiveness of unrelated BMTs. Information on becoming a marrow donor or initiating a search for a marrow donor can be obtained by calling their toll-free number. The NMDP sends an informative newsletter that includes a listing of all of the donor center locations and their phone numbers to each of its registered volunteers.

The American Bone Marrow Donor Registry is another organization involved in helping patients search for a donor. The Caitlin Raymond International Registry of Bone Marrow Donor Banks serves as a search-coordinating center. Their donor bank includes U.S. and international sources. They maintain one 800 number for those who want to be donors and another for those who want to initiate a search.

The International Bone Marrow Transplant Registry (IBMTR) is an organization that collects, organizes, and analyzes data about donor bone marrow transplants. They are strictly a research organization and are not involved in making donor matches. Their data is obtained from the many bone marrow transplant teams throughout the world. In the past, I received their statistical data on the number of transplants done annually, what diseases they were used to treat, and where they were done. A listing of all of the institutions throughout the world that perform donor transplants and participate in this registry can also be obtained.

A directory of BMT centers can be purchased for a small fee from the Oncology Nursing Society, which runs a BMT special-interest group. An updated 1994 directory is now available.

Another source for information on cancer and bone marrow transplantation is your public library or local book store. One of the best comprehensive books for cancer patients I have seen to date is

Everyone's Guide to Cancer Therapy: How Cancer Is Diagnosed, Treated, and Managed Day to Day by Malin Dollinger, M.D., Ernest H. Rosenbaum, M.D., and Greg Cable. It includes easy-to-understand descriptions of the many different kinds of cancer, including their common signs and symptoms, diagnostic tests, various stages, and treatments. The book also contains an informative chapter on bone marrow transplantation. (If you want more in-depth information on cancer and its staging, the American Cancer Society's *Cancer Manual*, which is written for medical professionals, includes a number of detailed tables listing the different staging systems and classifications used for each kind of cancer.)

Another excellent book, particularly for newly diagnosed patients, is *Diagnosis: Cancer Your Guide through the First Few Months* by Wendy Schlessel Harpham, M.D. It is easy to read and addresses many of the practical questions and concerns of most cancer patients. The author, in addition to being a physician, adds valuable advice and wisdom gained from her own experience as a cancer patient.

For breast cancer patients, there is an extremely informative book entitled *Breast Cancer: The Complete Guide* by Yashar Hirshaut, M.D., and Peter I. Pressman, M.D. The authors' clear, thorough explanations take women step by step from diagnosis to recovery. Included is a resource list from the National Alliance of Breast Cancer Organizations (NABCO) that provides a state-by-state listing of regional breast cancer support organizations.

A book that may be helpful for all female cancer patients, regardless of their kind of cancer, is *Beauty & Cancer* by Diane Doan Noyes and Peggy Mellody, R.N. This wonderful handbook is filled with practical suggestions to help women look and feel their best while coping with the side effects of cancer treatment. It includes information on wigs and headwraps (for those experiencing complete or partial hair loss), makeup tips, skin and nail care, clothing suggestions that address the body changes brought about by cancer treatment, and nutrition and exercise guides. (For women undergoing BMT, the sections that suggest kinds of clothing to wear when having a central venous catheter in your chest and types of headcovering to use when bald are particularly helpful.)

A fabulous, inspirational book for adult cancer patients is *Vital Signs: A Young Doctor's Struggle with Cancer* by Fitzhugh Mullan, M.D.

Although it does not deal with the topic of bone marrow transplantation, Dr. Mullan had a life-threatening illness and underwent radical treatment for cancer that involved prolonged hospitalization and recovery. His honest, moving story thoroughly explores the issues he faced while battling cancer in the prime of his life.

There are also some great sources of information for younger patients. *Teenagers Face to Face with Cancer,* by Karen Gravelle and Bertram A. John, describes the experiences of fifteen teens with cancer and one friend of a cancer patient. It is a candid and informative account of the special challenges faced by teens whose lives are touched by cancer.

An excellent book for children with cancer is *My Book for Kids with Cansur* by Jason Gaes. It is written by an 8-year-old boy who was diagnosed with a rare type of lymphoma when he was 6 years old. In his own words, misspellings and all, he describes his successful battle with cancer, shares his thoughts, and offers advice to other cancer patients. The book is illustrated by two of his brothers. It is an inspirational, authentic, and poignant work.

The National Cancer Institute also has some pamphlets available that may be helpful to younger patients and their families, such as *Help Yourself—Tips for Teenagers with Cancer, Young People with Cancer— A Handbook for Parents, Talking with Your Child about Cancer* (for children with cancer), and *When Someone in Your Family Has Cancer.*

Although there are very few books written specifically on bone marrow transplantation, in addition to Susan Stewart's book available from *BMT Newsletter,* there is another book entitled *Life's Blood* by Madeline Marget. *Life's Blood* includes the stories of a number of patients with life-threatening illnesses who underwent BMT under the care of Dr. Joel Rappeport, a renowned hematologist. Although the book contains a wealth of detailed information about BMT and the diseases it is used to treat, it can be difficult to read because of the depth of the information and of the heartrending negative outcomes experienced by many of the patients profiled. One other book, *Going for the Cure,* by Francesca M. Thompson, M.D., is available. It is unique in that it is an autobiographical account of the author's illness and experiences while undergoing an autologous BMT in 1989 for multiple myeloma. It is a very moving, easily read book.

Coping: Living with Cancer (published quarterly) is an excellent magazine written for cancer patients and their families. It contains helpful articles and information about other resources patients can utilize. Two examples are a booklet for children, titled *My Mommy Has Cancer*, by Carolyn Stearnes Parkinson, and a 2-hour video, called *Preparing for Bone Marrow Transplantation: One Patient's Perspective*, by Wayne St. James. The magazine offers a free catalog, containing books and videos that can be ordered, with each paid subscription.

Finally, for someone who wants really in-depth and recent information on cancer, bone marrow transplantation, or both, libraries at hospitals, colleges, and medical schools are additional reference sources. It is here that medical journal articles that detail the latest in research and treatment can be found. There are a number of oncology journals, and one journal that covers only BMT (entitled *Bone Marrow Transplantation*). Before you seek these sources, however, be aware that they can be difficult to read and understand due to complex medical explanations and terminology. They are written primarily for physicians and other health care professionals. Much can be gained by reading these journal articles, but take care not to let them create undue fear or frustration.

Sometimes you can also find new developments in the cancer field detailed in newsletters or publications distributed by your local hospital or oncology center. Occasionally, you will even hear about recent advances on news programs or read about them in the newspaper. Remember, however, that information in the media can sometimes be sensationalized to grab the public's attention and may contain inaccuracies. Watch the community services section of your local newspaper for information about local speakers who may be holding lectures or discussions on cancer-related topics of interest to you.

These are by no means all of the resources you can use to obtain information about cancer and its treatment, but I hope this section has given you some useful ideas about where to begin to expand your base of knowledge. You may find other resources available in your area or discover additional organizations or books that are helpful to you, perhaps even some that focus exclusively on BMT. As the number of bone marrow transplants grows each year, so does the need for easily obtainable information and support for prospective and surviving patients of this procedure.

Once you have collected data or are in the process of collecting data, you may wonder how you can possibly retain the many details about your disease or treatment that you read or are told. This can be particularly difficult if you are feeling tired, weak, or sick from your treatments. Here are some suggestions that may help.

- Read information in small bits at a time.
- When given verbal explanations, write things down immediately after they are told to you.
- Ask for many repetitions if you still don't grasp what's being said or are having trouble retaining it.
- Always question what you don't understand and ask for more simplistic explanations if the terms or complexity of the information seems overwhelming.
- Write down questions you want to ask your physician at your next office appointment or hospital visit. Write them down as soon as you think of them and have them readily accessible to refer to when the visit is made. Use a tape recorder if you have trouble writing due to treatment side effects.
- Above all, and it bears repeating, don't be afraid to ask questions and talk to your doctor about your concerns!

Some people still feel quite intimidated in the presence of doctors. Don't forget that, although physicians do have a great deal of specialized knowledge, they are human beings, too. The bottom line is that you are paying them for a service and not just for any service, but for one that involves your very life. Since you will need to be followed by an oncologist for the rest of your life, it is important to have a relationship that involves mutual respect. Communication and trust are also crucial to this relationship.

Just as we are all individuals with our own unique personalities and ways of relating to others, so too are physicians. You may find that you relate better to one doctor than another. Maybe it is because a doctor comes across as more caring or knowledgeable about you, or maybe it is just that you feel more comfortable in his or her presence. Whatever the reason, if you feel you have a better rapport with one particular physician, try to see him or her whenever possible.

If you are unhappy with your relationship with your doctor, are having adverse side effects, or don't feel confident about your treatment plan, speak up and discuss your concerns. Your doctor can't read your mind to know what you are thinking or feeling. You must tell him or her and ask questions. If you continue to be displeased after making several attempts to resolve what you find to be an unsatisfactory relationship, then, if possible, search for another oncologist in your area. Having cancer is hard enough without having to deal with the additional frustrations of feeling at odds with the source of your medical care.

(Information on the organizations and books mentioned in this section can be found in the appendix. Because it can be very helpful to have a good medical dictionary and prescription drug book on hand, several excellent reference books of this nature are also included.)

Dealing with Statistics

Sometime or another, you will no doubt be exposed to statistics about your disease. It may be because you have requested them, or they may be included in information about various treatment regimens, their side effects, or long-term outcomes. I have some words of advice to offer on this topic: Avoid being overly influenced by statistics. Sometimes, if they are favorable, they can give you an added boost or build confidence. If they are unfavorable, however, they can contribute to feelings of hopelessness and depression, particularly if you dwell on them.

The survival statistics cited at the time of my diagnosis were rather dismal using conventional chemotherapy regimens. You must keep in mind, as I did, that disease-free survival statistics help guide physicians by revealing which protocols of treatment have proven most effective in achieving remission and cure. Remember, though, that they do not say specifically how *you* will respond to a particular treatment.

Try to focus on the fact that even if the percentage is low, any survival statistic is made up of real people who are a part of this group because they have responded to this therapy with a maintained remission. I can't help but think of the words my mother used to say to bolster my morale in regard to the statistical information we were given. She'd say, "Even if the percentage rate of survival is low, someone has to be in that group and it might as well be you." And, of course, you have just as much right to be in that survival percentage as well!

I was confronted with the largest quantity of statistics at the transplant center when I went for my initial interview. Because physicians must inform you of every known potential complication of a specific treatment, this usually includes statistics detailing the percentage of patients who develop each complication. You will also be given an overall percentage of the effectiveness of bone marrow transplantation treatment in regard to your particular kind of cancer. This is usually given in terms of survival to specific points in time. It may be to an anniversary date that is 1, 2, 3, or even 5 years from the time of the transplant.

Statistics can help reinforce your physician's recommendation for BMT and may make you feel more comfortable in your decision to follow through with this treatment. It is very important for you to feel as confident as possible about the decisions made in regard to your care. This is especially true before undergoing a treatment as risky as bone marrow transplantation.

Although no one can predict the future, I felt, as did my physicians, that having a bone marrow transplant was the right treatment choice for me. That's not to say that it is always the best choice or even a treatment possibility for you. Only you, in conjunction with your doctor, can decide this. Learning the facts about bone marrow transplantation didn't take away my fear—sometimes it even made it worse—but it did give me confidence that I was involved in making an educated, informed decision.

One last word of caution about statistics. If you do research on your own, make sure statistical information is current and that it is truly applicable to your disease or treatment before you let it color any decisions you make. The field of medicine changes rapidly. I have seen several changes in the years since my own diagnosis and treatment. New procedures and medications can improve results and sometimes drastically alter old information. Always verify information with your oncologist before embracing it as true for you. Each patient is a unique individual, and even if information applies to your disease, it may be more or less significant when applied to your own particular case and medical history. When in doubt, ask your doctor.

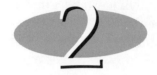

What Is a Bone Marrow Transplant?

There is a great deal of misunderstanding about bone marrow transplantation among the general public. These misconceptions were made quite evident to me when I was repeatedly asked, after my own transplant, about "my surgery" and where I was "cut open" to have the bone marrow inserted. I think that much of the confusion results from the fact that other organ transplants, such as a kidney, heart, or liver transplant, do require a surgical procedure. Therefore, most people naturally assume that a bone marrow transplant must involve cutting bones open to insert or remove marrow. In a bone marrow transplant, however, marrow is not transplanted surgically, but is instead transplanted by intravenous (I.V.) infusion into a patient's bloodstream (much like a blood transfusion).

Explaining the Procedure

To understand why someone might need a bone marrow transplant, it is necessary to understand what bone marrow is and what bodily function it performs. Bone marrow, which lies inside the cavities of bones, is a soft jelly-like spongy substance. It contains a system of blood vessels and connective tissue that holds together cells and fat. (When I saw samples of my own marrow, it looked just like thick, dark red blood.) Bone marrow's main function is to make new blood cells for the body. The most primitive cells in the marrow are the pluripotent stem cells. Stem cells can also be found in the peripheral bloodstream, only in much smaller quantities. It is from the pluripotent stem cells that each of the three main types of blood cells are made. These are the red blood cells, the white blood cells, and the platelets. The main function of the red cells is to carry oxygen from the lungs to body tissues, and then to transport carbon dioxide from body tissues back to the lungs to be exhaled. The white cells fight infection, and the platelets help blood clot.

Blood cells do not usually enter the bloodstream until they have gone through various stages and matured so they can function properly. Thus, cells in these various stages of maturity are normally found throughout the marrow. This can perhaps be better understood by viewing the evolution of the different cell lines. (See page 32.)

The most "marrow-rich" bones in the body, which contain the largest quantities of these stem cells, are the iliac (hip) bones in the pelvis, and the bone in the middle of the chest (the sternum). The site where marrow is most often removed from the body is at the pelvic bones. To obtain a marrow sample, a special needle is inserted through the skin and then down into the bone (after this tissue has been injected with medication to numb it). A syringe is attached to the needle, and the plunger is pulled back to withdraw a small portion of marrow. This procedure is called a bone marrow aspiration.

When a small piece of bone is removed in addition, it is called a bone marrow aspiration and biopsy. Layers of calcium are removed from the bone piece, and slices of it are then examined under a microscope. This gives a more precise view of how the marrow is actually functioning to make blood cells, as opposed to the more random sampling of cells obtained through aspiration.

When marrow is removed to be used for a bone marrow transplant, many aspirations of marrow are taken from either the patient or from a matched donor. This is to obtain a large enough quantity

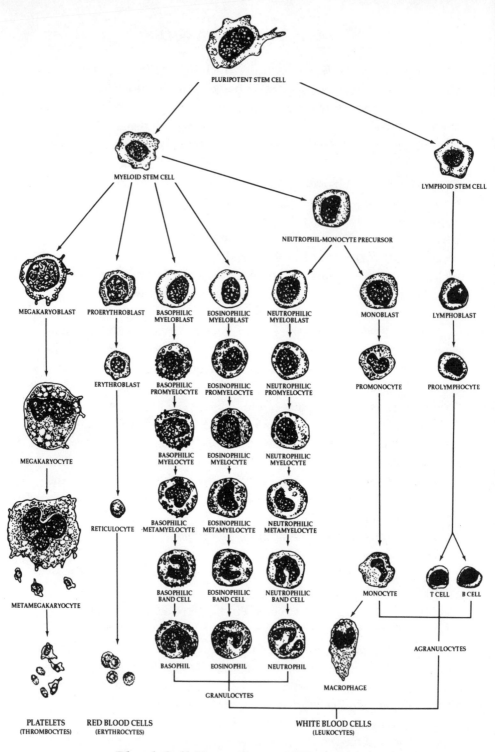

PLURIPOTENT STEM CELL

MYELOID STEM CELL

LYMPHOID STEM CELL

NEUTROPHIL-MONOCYTE PRECURSOR

MEGAKARYOBLAST

PROERYTHROBLAST

BASOPHILIC MYELOBLAST

EOSINOPHILIC MYELOBLAST

NEUTROPHILIC MYELOBLAST

MONOBLAST

LYMPHOBLAST

ERYTHROBLAST

BASOPHILIC PROMYELOCYTE

EOSINOPHILIC PROMYELOCYTE

NEUTROPHILIC PROMYELOCYTE

PROMONOCYTE

PROLYMPHOCYTE

MEGAKARYOCYTE

BASOPHILIC MYELOCYTE

EOSINOPHILIC MYELOCYTE

NEUTROPHILIC MYELOCYTE

RETICULOCYTE

BASOPHILIC METAMYELOCYTE

EOSINOPHILIC METAMYELOCYTE

NEUTROPHILIC METAMYELOCYTE

METAMEGAKARYOCYTE

BASOPHILIC BAND CELL

EOSINOPHILIC BAND CELL

NEUTROPHILIC BAND CELL

MONOCYTE

T CELL

B CELL

AGRANULOCYTES

BASOPHIL

EOSINOPHIL

NEUTROPHIL

MACROPHAGE

GRANULOCYTES

PLATELETS (THROMBOCYTES)

RED BLOOD CELLS (ERYTHROCYTES)

WHITE BLOOD CELLS (LEUKOCYTES)

Blood Cell Formation and Development

of stem cells so that blood production can be reestablished after the marrow is transplanted into the patient's bloodstream. The removal of a marrow for use in a bone marrow transplant is referred to as a bone marrow "harvest."

After reviewing the functions of bone marrow, you can under-

. . . .

Normal Values for Blood Cell Counts

White Blood Cell Count (WBC or Leukocytes)

Normal range for total count
(per cu. mm.)   5,000–10,000

Differential White Blood Cell Count

	Relative Values *(% of total number of white cells)*	*Absolute Values* *(number per cu.mm.)*
Granulocytes		
Neutrophils	50%–60%	3,000–7,000
Eosinophils	1%–4%	50–250
Basophils	0.5%–1%	25–100
Agranulocytes		
Lymphocytes	20%–40%	1,000–4,000
Monocytes	2%–6%	100–600

Red Blood Cell Count (RBC or Erythrocytes)

	Men	*Women*	*Children*
Normal range for total count (million/cu. mm.)	4.6–6.2	4.2–5.4	3.8–5.5

Hematocrit and Hemoglobin (H and H) Counts

	Men	*Women*	*Children*
Hematocrit (%/100 ml.)	40–54	37–47	31–43
Hemoglobin (gm./100 ml.)	14–18	12–16	11–16

Platelet Count (Thrombocytes)

Normal range for total count
(per cu. mm.)   150,000–400,000

. . . .

stand just how necessary properly functioning marrow is to keeping us alive and well. If the marrow becomes diseased or fails, blood cell production is altered or stops. Illness and death can rapidly follow without medical intervention.

The overwhelming majority of BMTs are used to treat cancer. Therefore, I will simply mention a few of the other diseases that bone marrow transplantation might be recommended for. BMT may be used to treat immune deficiency disorders, such as severe combined immunodeficiency syndrome (SCID) or Wiskott-Aldrich syndrome; cases of genetic or acquired bone marrow failure, such as aplastic anemia, Fanconi's anemia, thalassemia major, or osteopetrosis; or rare genetic metabolic diseases (referred to as the "storage diseases"), such as Gaucher's disease.

Bone marrow transplantation is most often used in the treatment of certain types of cancers that arise from the blood-making cells of the bone marrow. These diseases either have no other curative treatment options or are difficult to eradicate with conventional treat-

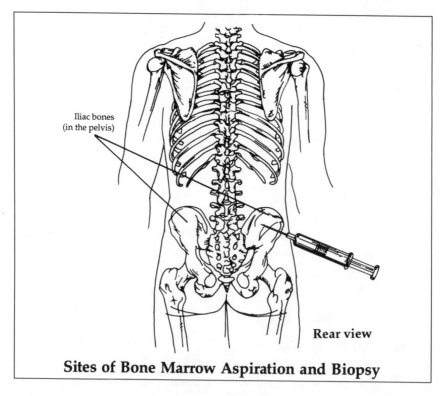

Iliac bones
(in the pelvis)

Rear view

Sites of Bone Marrow Aspiration and Biopsy

ments. This is because the doses of chemotherapy and/or radiation that are needed to destroy the cancer cells and abnormal stem cells prevalent with these diseases are so high that they would destroy healthy blood-making cells as well. (Bone marrow cells, even normal ones, are especially sensitive to the effects of high-dose chemotherapy and radiation.) When bone marrow is transplanted after cancer treatment, however, this not only makes the use of extremely high-dose therapy possible, but also allows for the replacement of diseased marrow with healthy marrow.

Patients who have cancer originating in other parts of their bodies may also need aggressive anticancer therapy to eradicate cancer cells. If such treatment is used, their healthy bone marrow would most likely be destroyed as a side effect. Therefore, if high-dose anticancer treatment is necessary, these patients also need a bone marrow transplant, not specifically as a treatment for the cancer itself, but as a "rescue" procedure to replace destroyed marrow. These patients use a portion of their own marrow, which is removed and stored prior to treatment, for the transplant. Essentially, the major advantage BMT has over conventional treatment is that physicians can use more aggressive anticancer treatments without concern for the lethal side effects they have on normal marrow, because marrow is transplanted after treatment (with either donor marrow or with a portion of a patient's own marrow).

Before the actual marrow transplant takes place, a course of intensive high-dose chemotherapy or chemotherapy and total body irradiation (TBI) is given. This pretransplant, anticancer therapy is called the preparative regimen or conditioning regimen (further explained in chapter 5). Whether a patient receives chemotherapy or a combination of chemotherapy and radiation depends on the underlying disease and what protocols of treatment are currently being used at the center where the patient is treated.

Chemotherapy drugs, as well as virtually all other I.V. medications, are given to BMT patients through a catheter (a flexible tube) that is surgically inserted into a large vein near the collarbone prior to treatment. These central venous (vein) catheters (CVCs) are usually referred to by their brand name, such as a Hickman catheter, a Groshong catheter, or a Broviac catheter (a smaller diameter catheter used for children and some adults). If a patient does not have a CVC already in place from prior therapy, one is inserted at the transplant center soon after admission. There are several advantages to having this kind of I.V. device instead of the usual kind of catheter that is inserted into a hand or arm vein. A CVC can remain in place for an extended period of time, saves the patient from numerous "sticks" in the arms because blood specimens can be drawn from it, and helps prevent damage to vein walls from toxic medications because it is inserted into a large vein with greater blood flow.

Once the preparative regimen is finished, there are 1 to 2 days of rest before the actual transplant takes place. This is to ensure that any residual effects from the treatment will not destroy any of the new marrow that is given. On the day of the transplant, either the patient's own (previously removed) marrow, or marrow taken from a donor, is given intravenously (through the central venous catheter) in the patient's hospital room. If a donor's marrow is used, it is usually contained in an I.V. bag and looks similar to a big bag of blood. It is infused by slow intravenous drip into the patient's blood-

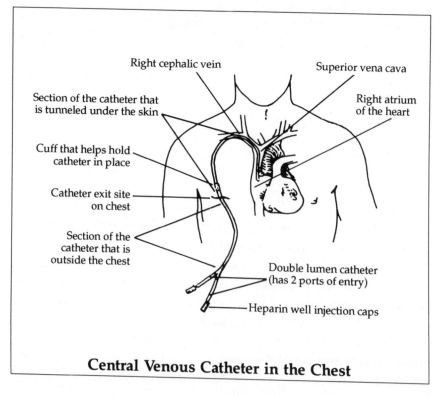

Central Venous Catheter in the Chest

stream, much like a blood transfusion. If a patient's marrow is used, it is often contained in a syringe (although sometimes it is also in an I.V. bag). Depending on which is used, it is either slowly injected or dripped into the patient's bloodstream.

The transplanted marrow eventually migrates from the bloodstream to the sites in the bones where it normally resides. It will then, hopefully, begin to grow and produce healthy new blood cells. When it begins to do this, the marrow is said to have "engrafted." It usually takes 2 to 4 weeks, after the transplant, for the new marrow to produce sufficient numbers of white blood cells, red blood cells, and platelets.

Bone marrow transplantation is often explained using the analogy of planting seeds in a garden and then waiting for them to grow. The goal is to keep the patient alive with supportive care, and to try and prevent complications from occurring, until the transplanted marrow begins to "grow" and produce enough blood cells to sustain and protect his or her body.

The Different Types of Transplants

There are two main types of transplant: those that use a patient's own marrow and those that use a donor's marrow. Different terms are used to describe the transplant depending upon the source of the marrow. An *allogeneic* transplant is one that uses marrow from a matched donor. The donor is usually related to the patient (most often a sibling), but does not have to be. A *syngeneic* transplant is one that uses marrow from an identical twin, and an *autologous* transplant is one that uses a patient's own marrow for his or her transplant. A peripheral stem cell transplant is a form of autologous transplant, in which stem cells from the peripheral bloodstream are used. The type of transplant a doctor recommends depends on several factors. These include the kind and extent of cancer a patient has, if donor marrow offers a higher chance for disease-free survival, and whether the patient has an available matched donor.

If a patient is going to have an autologous transplant, some of his or her own stem cells must be removed before the preparative regimen is given. This can be done in two ways. Marrow can be removed by aspiration from the iliac bones in a procedure that is basically the same as that used for a matched donor. The second way this can be done is through peripheral stem cell harvesting. In a process called apheresis, blood is withdrawn through an I.V. catheter and circulated through a cell-separating machine. Components in the blood that are wanted (in this case, stem cells) are extracted, while unneeded blood components are returned to the patient through another I.V. line. An advantage of this procedure is that it does not require anesthesia. It can also be done on an outpatient basis, although it may require as many as three or more separate trips to the hospital to obtain the desired quantity of stem cells that need to be harvested. This is because the concentration of stem cells in the peripheral blood is 10 to 100 times less than that in the bone marrow.

Sometimes agents called growth factors are used to increase the production of blood cells prior to harvesting. Colony-stimulating factors (CSFs), a category of growth factors, are proteins that specifically stimulate the production and growth of certain kinds of blood cells. Two that may be used to improve white blood cell production are G-CSF (granulocyte colony-stimulating factor) and GM-CSF (granulocyte-macrophage colony-stimulating factor). CSFs are also sometimes used after certain types of transplants to hasten the return of blood counts. Bringing about a more rapid return of particular kinds of white blood cells may reduce the patient's risk of post-transplant infection.

Although it has been proposed by some researchers that peripheral blood may provide a more cancer-free source for stem cells, particularly if a patient is known to have cancer in his or her bone marrow, this is debated by others. It does, however, provide another source for stem cells that can be used alone or in conjunction with harvested bone marrow to increase the quantity given back to the patient after the preparative regimen.

Careful consideration is given in determining when the bone marrow or peripheral stem cell harvesting should be done. It depends largely on the status of the patient's health, his or her tumor burden, and when the transplant is scheduled. Ideally, it should be removed when the patient is in remission so there are no or few cancer cells present. Depending on the patient's disease, marrow may be treated with a chemotherapy agent (such as 4HC) or with other methods to purge (remove) any existing cancer cells before it is preserved and frozen. It is filtered through a stainless steel screen to remove small bone fragments and break up clumps of cells. The cells are then combined with a preservative to keep them alive while they are frozen. One preservative, Dimethyl sulfoxide (DMSO), emits a strong, persistent garlic-like smell. Measures to mask this odor may be employed. Marrow may be stored for 3 or more years, depending on the method of preservation. Stronger doses of anticancer agents can be used on this marrow because it is treated outside the patient's body, although care must be taken not to damage too many normal cells in the process.

One of the other methods used by some centers to purge marrow of cancer cells is through the use of monoclonal antibodies. (An antibody is a protein made by the body's immune system to inactivate a specific foreign substance. Substances that can initiate this response are called antigens.) Monoclonal antibodies are manufactured in a laboratory and, when used in this case, are "programmed" to attach to tumor antigens. They can interfere with a cancer cell's growth factors; carry anticancer drugs, toxins, or radioactive particles into a cancer cell to destroy it; mark tumors for destruction when combined with other agents; or carry microscopic metallic beads to tumors so they can be removed when passed over a magnetic field.

Monoclonal antibodies can also be used to target other types of cells. They are sometimes used to purge T lymphocytes from donor marrow to try to prevent or minimize a particular post-transplant complication called graft-versus-host disease (see chapter 3 for further explanation). Graft-versus-host disease (GVHD) occurs when immune cells in the transplanted marrow, certain T lymphocytes, launch an attack on body tissues of the recipient because they are recognized as foreign. For this reason, if a patient's disease warrants the use of donor marrow, human leukocyte antigen (HLA) testing must be done on blood samples taken from both a patient and potential donor to determine their tissues' compatibility.

HLA antigens, located at certain sites (the histo-compatible genetic areas found on chromosome six) on the surface of white blood cells, play an important role in our body's immune response to foreign substances. The antigens that have been identified as being the most important in determining whether a rejection reaction will occur between two people's tissues are those located at the HLA-A, HLA-B, and HLA-DR sites. At each of these sites, we have 2 antigens. We inherit 1 from each parent. Although there are many different types of antigens known, which can combine genetically in many different ways, the odds of having a brother or sister match your particular combination of HLA antigens are approximately 1 in 4. This is because we tend to inherit the antigens at these 3 sites together in a group, which is called a haplotype. This means that we generally have 1 haplotype that is similar to 1 of the 2 our mother has and 1 haplotype that is similar to 1 of the 2 our father has.

As a result, the best chance of finding a match among these 6 antigens is between siblings, although parents and other closely related people are often tested to determine their compatibility as well. Certain haplotypes are more common among the general population than others. Thus, according to the NMDP the odds of matching an unrelated individual are between 1 and 100 and 1 and 1 million, depending on your particular antigen types. Because these HLA antigens are inherited, your ethnic background can play a significant role in your ability to find an unrelated donor if a related donor does not exist.

If all three of these pairs of another person's antigens match yours, another test, called a mixed lymphocyte culture (MLC), is then done to further evaluate the match. (It is used to better define the HLA-D antigen.) Samples of the recipient and potential donor lymphocytes are mixed and cultured. Lab testing is performed, utilizing a radioactive substance to "tag" cells to determine whether they react against one another. If there is a substantial reaction, the donor may be deemed unsuitable. If they don't react negatively, it is said to be a "perfect match." A perfect match really only exists, however, between identical twins (because they are genetically identical). In an allogeneic transplant, even in the case of a 6-antigen match, there are still often minor incompatibilities because the donor and recipient are not genetically identical. This is evidenced by the fact that not all 6-antigen matches work out successfully in reality. As a matter of fact, graft-versus-host disease is not all that uncommon following allogeneic bone marrow transplants. Because it is more likely, however, that a related donor will match in minor ways as well, a related 6-antigen match is considered safer than an unrelated 6-antigen match. This still does not guarantee that the transplant will be successful, just that the odds are higher that severe immune rejection problems will not occur.

Finally, note that bone marrow transplants differ from other organ transplants in that a 6-antigen match is almost always essential before an allogeneic bone marrow transplant is undertaken. (Once in a while a transplant will be tried using a donor with a lesser match, particularly when there are absolutely no other potentially

. . . .

Inheritance of HLA Antigens

PARENT'S ANTIGENS*

Mother   **Father**

Haplotype 1	Haplotype 2	Haplotype 1	Haplotype 2
A	B	C	D

POSSIBLE COMBINATIONS OF ANTIGENS IN CHILDREN**

Child 1		**Child 2**		**Child 3**		**Child 4**	
A	C	A	D	B	C	B	D

*Each Haplotype consists of one HLA-A, one HLA-B, and one HLA-DR antigen. To simplify the explanation, a single letter has been used to represent the sets. (Another HLA antigen [HLA-C] lies between HLA-A and HLA-B. If HLA-A and HLA-B are identical, HLA-C is generally identical, too.)

**Although the odds of matching a sibling are 1 in 4, the number of siblings you have does not in any way guarantee or rule out the possibility of a match. You may have many siblings, but be the only one who inherited one of the above combinations. On the other hand, you may only have one sibling and, just by chance, both of you could have inherited the same combination of HLA antigens.

. . . .

curative treatment options.) This extremely close antigen match is advocated because allogeneic BMT involves actually transplanting a new immune system into someone's body, not just suppressing an existing one to prevent a "foreign" organ from being rejected. Other organ transplants, such as kidney transplants, are often successful with a less than perfect match.

What a Donor Can Expect

In addition to the almost perfect compatibility needed between a donor's and recipient's HLA type, bone marrow transplant donation differs from other organ transplants in that the donor does not permanently lose the organ given to the recipient. Only a small portion of the donor's marrow is removed, approximately 3% to 5%. The bone marrow that is removed replenishes itself within a matter of weeks. During this time the donor may be asked to take an iron supplement. Donors usually donate a few units of their own blood ahead of time, which are then given back to them shortly after the bone marrow harvest takes place.

The first step any potential donor undergoes is to have blood drawn to verify that his or her HLA type and the patient's are compatible. After this is confirmed, many additional tubes of blood are drawn to verify the donor's health and check other factors that are pertinent to the transplant, such as the presence of antibodies indicative of past infections.

The donor and recipient *do not* need to have the same blood type. This is because the recipient's immune system is destroyed by the preparative regimen, so he or she should no longer have antibodies against foreign blood types. (The major blood types are A, B, AB, and O.) If blood types differ, the recipient will convert to the donor's blood type after the transplant.

In addition to blood testing, donors undergo a thorough physical, a chest X ray, an EKG (electrocardiogram), and have a complete health history taken. When a related donor is used, this testing usually takes place at the transplant center where the patient is to be admitted. When an unrelated donor is used, the testing is usually done at the authorized bone marrow collection site that is closest to the donor's home. Donation procedures are explained, and pretransplant counseling is given to all prospective donors.

Once preliminary tests are completed and found to be satisfactory, the donor waits for word on when the marrow removal procedure will occur. Until this time, and particularly once the recipient begins the pretransplant regimen, donors are asked not to engage in any hazardous activities. This is for obvious reasons because, once the patient's bone marrow is destroyed, he or she is totally dependent on the donor's marrow to recover.

The donor is admitted to the hospital either the night before or the morning of the procedure. He or she has an intravenous line inserted just like any other surgical patient. In the Operating Room, either general anesthesia or a spinal block is used to prevent the donor from experiencing pain as the marrow is withdrawn. The procedure is virtually the same as that described at the beginning of this chapter for a bone marrow aspiration, except that there are usually 2 to 4 removal site punctures made in the iliac bones above each buttock.

Multiple "pulls" (attaching and drawing back the syringe to remove marrow) are made at each puncture site, perhaps as many as 20 to 30. Usually 1 to 2 pints of marrow are removed from the donor. The actual quantity harvested, however, depends on a number of factors, such as patient size, donor size, and the concentration and composition of cells in the donor's marrow.

A team effort is employed by the physician and his or her assistants to remove this marrow as expeditiously as possible to decrease the time a donor remains under anesthesia. The donor is monitored by a member of the anesthesia team throughout the procedure just as would occur with any other surgical procedure.

Once the desired quantity of marrow is harvested, pressure is held over each of the removal sites for approximately 5 minutes, after which a sterile dressing is applied. The patient is then transferred to the Post-Anesthesia Care Unit (PACU), formerly called the Recovery Room, until the effects of the anesthesia have worn off. From there, the donor is sent back to his or her regular hospital room and usually remains there overnight to be monitored until discharge the next morning.

Pain medication is prescribed as needed for soreness at the puncture sites. Usually, regular Tylenol is adequate to relieve this discomfort. Most of the soreness disappears within a week or two and donors often resume their normal schedule of activities a few days after the procedure. Donors may experience some tiredness until their marrow replaces the quantity that was removed.

There is relatively low risk associated with bone marrow donation, particularly when compared to other organ donation, and complications are extremely infrequent. The main risks are possible infection and/or bleeding at the puncture sites, and those risks associated with anesthesia.

The following paragraphs were written by my bone marrow donor. They will give you a better understanding of what an actual donor may experience physically and emotionally.

. . . .

A Donor's Message

"Your sister has leukemia and may die." If you are the family member or friend of a cancer patient for whom bone marrow transplantation is recommended, you too may have heard words similar to these, as I did in 1989. I experienced feelings of anger, sorrow, and downright helplessness. Then my whole family was tissue-typed, using the HLA test, to determine if a good enough match existed for my sister to receive a related-donor transplant. It was determined that I was a perfect match! Suddenly my sister's life depended on *me*. Gone was the feeling of helplessness, because I could indeed make a tangible contribution to her cure, but that feeling was replaced by others that were much more complicated.

Naturally, everyone in my family assumed that I would donate bone marrow for my sister. And it was true, as soon as we found out about the match, I assured family and doctors alike that I was ready and willing. In the end, what choice did I really have? Without the transplant she would have probably died. This contributed greatly to feelings of pressure, stress, and fear.

Being a donor is a tremendous responsibility, one that I felt keenly throughout the whole process leading up to the transplant. What if the transplant didn't work? Would I be responsible for that, too? The doctors who counseled me cautioned against blaming myself if the procedure was not successful. Fortunately, I never had to find out how I would have reacted because my sister's transplant was a resounding success!

Many people I spoke with prior to the procedure assumed that being a bone marrow donor would be very painful. I had endured health problems of my own in the past, including a history of two kidney transplants, so I was familiar with being hospitalized for surgical procedures. To tell the truth, the procedure was not as painful as I thought it might be. Sure I was stiff and sore afterward, but there was no sharp piercing pain. Each person reacts differently to physical discomfort, however, and our own personal tolerance level depends on many things.

Once the anesthesia wore off, I found that the best thing for me to do was to keep moving. My sister and I had rooms located right next to each other, and I remember getting up during the night to visit with her and walk around the transplant floor. I spent a total of approximately 2 days time in the hospital—I checked in during the afternoon of Day 1, three pints of my bone marrow were harvested the morning of Day 2, and I was discharged the morning of Day 3.

I went home on a Thursday and went back to work on Monday. I did tire more easily at first and sat on a pillow for about a week because I was still sore. I also took iron tablets for approximately 2 months to help rebuild my bone marrow, but I had absolutely no lasting ill effects from the harvesting procedure.

There is now a bond between my sister and me that goes beyond that of normal family ties. She will carry my bone marrow within her for the rest of her life. I am extremely proud of the way she courageously fought this battle for her life, and I am proud that I turned out to be the secret weapon that clinched her victory.

We all have the power to give that most precious of gifts to our fellow human beings—a new lease on life. Please be an organ donor. Have it so noted on your driver's license and tell family members of your decision in case you can't speak for yourself. If you have a living will, include your wish to be an organ donor. My sister and I are living full lives today because of kidney and bone marrow donations. This is truly one of the most tangible examples of love for a fellow human being. Life—pass it on!

Cancers BMT May Be Used to Treat

Bone marrow transplants are perhaps best known for their use in the treatment of leukemia. Leukemia is actually a category of a group of cancers that originate in the blood-forming cells of the body. It is generally characterized by the unregulated production of abnormal white blood cells. White cells are called leukocytes and -emia is an ending referring to the blood, hence the name leukemia for the disease. (Despite its name, in rare cases, leukemia can also involve the production of abnormal red blood cells and/or platelets.) Although leukemic cells, as well as cancer cells in general, do not divide more rapidly than normal cells, because they don't differentiate and mature like noncancerous cells, they have an advantage over normal cells.

The overabundance of abnormal white blood cells that are typically produced in leukemia eventually crowd out other normal marrow cells and symptoms of infection, bleeding, and anemia develop. These symptoms may include fevers, recurrent colds or other infections, shortness of breath, weakness, chronic fatigue, swollen gums, pale complexion, prolonged or unstoppable bleeding (perhaps evident in the form of nose bleeds, gum bleeding with dental procedures, or increased menstrual bleeding in women), excessive bruising, a pinpoint red skin rash (called petechiae), pain in bones or joints, and/or swelling of lymph nodes or body organs (such as the spleen).

To better understand leukemia and its various types, it is helpful to have a basic understanding of the different kinds of white blood cells. White blood cells are divided into 2 groups, the granulocytes and the agranulocytes. There are 3 types of granulocytes (neutrophils, eosinophils, and basophils) and 2 types of agranulocytes (monocytes and lymphocytes). Granulocytes derive their name from the small, grainlike particles, called granules, that are present in their cells. Agranulocytes do not have these particles. In addition to being formed in the bone marrow, agranulocytes can also be produced from lymphoid tissue in the spleen, tonsils, and lymph nodes.

Neutrophils are the most numerous and important kind of granulocyte because they defend against bacterial infection. They are often just called "polys" (because their nucleus consists of several parts). The function of eosinophils and basophils is less clearly understood.

Eosinophils are believed to combat certain parasitic infections and the allergens that cause allergies. Basophils are believed to be involved in allergic reactions and are sometimes found in increased numbers in association with tissue that is chronically inflamed or is in the process of healing.

Monocytes, the largest of the white blood cells, serve as the body's second line of defense against infection. They clear the body of microorganisms by "ingesting" them. Lymphocytes are small, mobile white blood cells that are important in regulating both the production of antibodies and our immune response to foreign substances. There are two types of lymphocytes, T cells and B cells. The T cells, made in the bone marrow and "matured" by the thymus gland when we're young, destroy foreign substances (those that are not recognized as part of our own body). T cells are sometimes referred to as "killer T cells." The B cells, made in the bone marrow, spleen, and lymph nodes, are involved in the production of antibodies. When B cells come into contact with a particular foreign antigen, they turn into plasma cells and produce antibodies against it. This provides us with immunity because these foreign antigens are "remembered." They will initiate an immune response if we are exposed to them again in the future.

Leukemias are classified not only according to which type of blood cell is responsible for producing the cancerous cells but also according to the maturity of the malignant cells. If the cells produced are immature, resulting in a rapid progression of the disease symptoms, then it is called acute leukemia. If the cancer cells produced are more mature, resulting in a slower progression of the disease, then it is called chronic leukemia.

Because the initial symptoms of leukemia can be vague and similar to those of common illnesses, they may be overlooked by the patient, or even the physician, in the earlier stages of the disease. I attributed the chest and back pain I had to sore muscles. I now know that this pain resulted from the excessive number of leukemia cells that were being "packed" into my sternum and ribs. I also didn't realize that the recurrent sties I had on my eyelids (small, painful bumps caused by bacterial infection) were the result of my body's decreased ability to fight infection.

Many times, just as in my case, leukemia is actually discovered "by accident" through a blood test done for some other purpose, such as for a routine physical or as part of presurgical testing. This is particularly true for those with chronic leukemia. Their symptoms are generally even more vague and are often nonexistent in the early stages.

Leukemia is diagnosed through blood tests and confirmed by a bone marrow aspiration and biopsy. The leukemias are basically divided into those that originate in lymphocytes (the lymphocytic leukemias) and those that do not (the myelogenous leukemias). Myelogenous means "originating in marrow" and includes all the leukemias that arise from the granulocytes, monocytes, red blood cells, or platelets. The 4 main types of leukemia are acute lymphocytic leukemia (ALL), acute myelogenous leukemia (AML), chronic lymphocytic leukemia (CLL), and chronic myelogenous leukemia (CML). Acute myelogenous leukemia is also sometimes referred to as acute nonlymphocytic leukemia (ANLL).

Although there are 7 basic subtypes of AML, there are a number of other general terms that are often used interchangeably with acute myelogenous leukemia, such as acute granulocytic leukemia, acute myelocytic leukemia, and acute myeloblastic leukemia. ALL may also be referred to as acute lymphoblastic leukemia, and CML may also be referred to as chronic granulocytic leukemia or chronic myelocytic leukemia. Having your disease referred to by a variety of names can be very confusing, particularly at first, until you come to understand the different cell lines and recognize why these various descriptions are used. (Refer back to the illustration on page 32.)

Although some people think of acute leukemia as only a childhood disease, statistically, more adults are diagnosed each year with acute leukemia than children. ALL is much more common in children, whereas AML is more common in adults. Just like AML, ALL has a number of different types. Initial treatment for the acute leukemias, called "induction chemotherapy," involves the administration of various chemotherapy drugs that are aimed at inducing a remission. A "complete" remission is one in which there are no cancer cells detected after treatment. Because undetected cancer cells are often still present, however, follow-up treatment called "consolidation chemotherapy," and sometimes even "maintenance chemotherapy," is given. Treatment may also include the administration of chemotherapy and/or radiation to the central nervous system, if leukemic cells are present in the brain and spinal cord (which is more likely in ALL).

Although improvements in treatment have led to higher rates of complete remission and cure, especially for children under 15 years of age with certain types of ALL, the risk for relapse (a return of the cancer) can still be relatively high for many acute leukemia patients following conventional treatments. (This is because all of the abnormal stem cells causing the cancer cannot generally be eliminated.) If a relapse is likely to occur, if it has already occurred, or if an initial complete remission has never been achieved from induction chemotherapy, extremely high doses of anticancer treatment, followed by bone marrow transplantation, may be the best or only treatment that can offer a patient the chance for long-term survival. An allogeneic transplant is usually the preferred type of transplant for acute leukemia patients. If there is no available matched donor, however, an autologous transplant may be recommended. Improvements in eliminating cancer cells from harvested marrow have made this a potentially curative treatment option today as well.

BMT is also used as a treatment for the chronic leukemias, particularly for CML. CML is distinguished by the presence of something called the Philadelphia chromosome. This is a genetic abnormality that involves a break and subsequent recombination of 2 chromosomes (the 9th and 22d) to create a new, abnormal diseased cell. (In rare cases, the Philadelphia chromosome can also be present in ALL.) Although there are few, if any, symptoms early in the course of the disease, an enlarged spleen can be one early symptom. Patients with an enlarged spleen may be aware of what seems to be a mass on the left upper side of their abdomen. Eventually, CML patients usually progress from this chronic phase of the disease to an acute phase of the disease (called a "blast crisis"). When this happens, the disease is often not very responsive to treatment. Even if remission can be attained, it usually tends not to last long.

Although there are medications such as busulfan, hydroxyurea, and interferon that can be effective in controlling CML while it is in the chronic phase, this disease is generally considered to be curable only with an allogeneic BMT. BMT has been found to be the most successful when performed relatively early during the chronic phase of the disease (within a year or so after diagnosis). Although autologous BMTs have not been very successful in eradicating CML in the past, there are some current clinical trials utilizing this type of transplant for CML patients.

The other type of chronic leukemia, CLL, rarely occurs in younger persons. The average age of those diagnosed with this form of leukemia is 65. Patients may live for many years before the disease progresses and symptoms such as anemia, bleeding, recurrent infections, and/or swollen lymph nodes emerge. Chemotherapy is often not initiated until symptoms such as these appear. Conventional treatment is generally only palliative (serving to reduce symptoms), not curative. The only potentially curative treatment, at present, is considered to be allogeneic BMT. Because patients are usually older when diagnosed with this disease, however, BMT is an infrequent treatment for this type of leukemia because older age predisposes patients to increased complications.

No discussion of leukemia would be complete without mentioning myelodysplastic syndrome (MDS). This is the name given to a group of blood disorders that are often referred to as preleukemia, because patients can progress from one subtype to another and eventually develop acute myelogenous leukemia (AML). MDS is characterized by the abnormal production of a wide variety of different types of blood cells, such as granulocytes, platelets, and erythrocytes. Chromosomal abnormalities in the cancer cells are relatively common.

MDS most often appears in persons over 60 years of age, but can occasionally occur in younger persons as well. In some cases it is a "secondary cancer," meaning one that occurs after previous treatment for a different kind of cancer. Patients with MDS may begin chemotherapy shortly after diagnosis, or they may be watched closely for a number of weeks or months before treatment is initiated. During this time, supportive therapies, such as blood transfusions, are administered as needed. Depending on the patient's age and physical condition, bone marrow transplantation may be recommended for those with HLA-matched donors.

Another kind of bone marrow cancer is multiple myeloma. This cancer differs from leukemia in that it originates in plasma cells. Plasma cells are made from a type of white blood cell called a B lymphocyte. When B lymphocytes come into contact with particular foreign substances, they change into antibody-producing plasma cells. Multiple myeloma is diagnosed through blood, urine, and bone marrow tests. Malignant plasma cells produce large quantities of abnormal immunoglobulins (certain types of antibodies that can be detected in the blood—it's known as the M component or M spike). Fragments of these immunoglobulins are excreted in the urine as Bence Jones proteins, which can lead to kidney failure.

Staging (medical testing to determine the extent of the cancer) is done upon diagnosis. This may include X rays, bone scans, CT (computerized tomography) scans, and/or MRIs (magnetic resonance imaging) to detect bone tumors or "holes" in the patient's skeleton caused by these tumors. The disease is classified as either Stage I, II, or III (depending on the quantity of abnormal cells present). It is also further classified into 2 subtypes according to how the kidneys are functioning (Subtype A indicates that kidney function is relatively normal, and Subtype B indicates signs of kidney failure.)

Symptoms of the disease may include back, chest, or bone pain; bone fractures; bleeding; anemia (characterized by weakness, fatigue, pale skin color, and shortness of breath); infections (such as pneumonia); high blood calcium levels; kidney failure; and neurological problems caused by tumors pressing on nerves. Treatment consists mainly of chemotherapy, although sometimes radiation therapy may be used for pain control. At present, bone marrow transplantation is considered the only potentially curative treatment. Either allogeneic or autologous transplantation may be tried depending on the patient's circumstances. Peripheral stem cell harvesting may also accompany an autologous transplant.

The purpose of BMT is to destroy the cancerous plasma cells along with the cells that they arise from. However, myeloma cells can be difficult to eradicate completely, even with high-dose therapy. And, in the case of an autologous transplant, myeloma cells can be difficult to remove completely from marrow that is to be reinfused into the patient. Even without a cure, BMT may bring about a more prolonged remission from the disease. But BMT is not a common treatment for this disease because the average age of those diagnosed with multiple myeloma is approximately 60.

Lymphoma is the general name for the group of diseases that

have cancerous cells originating in the lymphatic system. This system of the body is made up of lymph, lymph vessels, lymph nodes, the tonsils, the thymus gland, and the spleen. Lymph is a clear, colorless fluid that consists of proteins and water. The primary way it differs from blood is that it does not contain red blood cells. The lymphatic system functions to collect and drain the lymph fluid that has escaped from blood vessels into tissue spaces. It is circulated through lymph vessels and filtered of foreign matter by lymph nodes (which produce lymphocytes and monocytes) before it reenters the bloodstream. The lymphatic system plays an important role in our immune system.

The two most common types of lymphoma are Hodgkin's disease and non-Hodgkin's lymphoma. Hodgkin's disease (HD) derives its name from Thomas Hodgkin, the British physician who first described this disease in 1832. The cancerous cell in HD is a giant cell referred to as a Reed-Sternberg cell. The type of HD is determined by microscopic examination of these tumor cells. A unique characteristic of HD is that it tends to spread from one group of lymph nodes to the next in a rather orderly fashion.

The disease is divided into 4 basic stages. Stage I denotes the involvement of only one lymph node region, while Stage IV denotes widespread disease. The stage is determined by some or all of the following procedures: blood tests; bone marrow aspiration and biopsy; chest and bone X rays; CT scans of the chest, abdomen, and pelvis; a gallium scan (a test that is done by injecting radioactive particles into the bloodstream followed by the taking of pictures with a machine that scans body tissues); MRIs; lymphangiography (a test that involves injecting a contrast dye into an area of the feet—this dye then spreads into the lymphatic system and follow-up X rays are taken); and/or laparotomy (a surgical exploration of the abdomen). This surgical procedure may involve removing the spleen (splenectomy) and/or abdominal nodes and liver tissue for biopsy. It is often referred to as a "staging laparotomy."

Some of the symptoms of HD are painless swellings of lymph nodes in the neck or under the arms, fevers, intense itching (such as on the soles of the feet), loss of weight, chills, night sweats, shortness of breath, cough, and discomfort in the chest. Localized tumors are treated with radiation therapy, and chemotherapy is used for more extensive disease. Because HD is often cured with conventional therapy, particularly in its early stages, BMT is not a common treatment. But for those who have been treated with a number of different regimens and have either not obtained a remission, or who continue to have relapses and progressive disease, BMT may be the only real hope for a cure.

Autologous BMT is the most common type of transplant for HD patients. The preparative regimen, administered prior to the reinfusion of the patient's harvested marrow, often consists of only high-dose combination chemotherapy. Total body irradiation does not usually accompany the chemotherapy, because most of these patients have already received the most radiation therapy they can have safely. Although autologous BMT is the norm, allogeneic BMT may be attempted for patients who have a matched donor and extensive disease that has infiltrated the bone marrow.

Non-Hodgkin's lymphoma occurs more commonly than HD, and is actually a grouping for a number of different types of cancer of the lymphatic system. These cancers range from those that are acute and rapidly growing to those that are slow-growing (indolent) and chronic in nature. There are many different subgroups that have been identified in this disease. As you may remember, there are 2 different kinds of lymphocytes, B cells and T cells. The vast majority of lymphomas are believed to originate from B cells.

Non-Hodgkin's lymphoma does not have the orderly way of spreading from node to adjacent node that HD does, and it can originate or spread anywhere in the body that lymphocytes are found. Its symptoms can be quite vague and insidious, like those of some of the other cancers. People with lymphoma often have advanced disease at the time of diagnosis, although they may still feel rather well. The disease may be found "by accident," as a result of routine tests, or after individuals discover an enlarged lymph node that prompts them to see their physician.

There are different ways of classifying non-Hodgkin's lymphomas depending on the cell type, where the malignant cells are located, how quickly they grow, and what kind of symptoms the patient is experiencing. There are 3 different "grades" (low, intermediate, and high), as well as 4 different stages (Stages I through IV). Non-Hodgkin's lymphomas are further differentiated by the absence or presence of certain symptoms, which are classified as "A" or "B" accordingly. "B" symptoms include such things as fever, night sweats, and/or weight loss. Patients without these fall into the "A" category. (These classifications are also used in Hodgkin's disease.)

Additional symptoms of non-Hodgkin's lymphoma may be abdominal discomfort, changes in bowel habits, sinus problems, sore throat, cough, difficulty swallowing, headaches, and/or anemia. Diagnosis is made through the surgical removal and biopsy of involved lymph nodes and is accompanied by some or all of the following tests: bone marrow biopsy, chest X ray, CT scans, gallium scanning, lymphangiogram, MRI scanning, or even a spinal tap (if neurological involvement is suspected).

As in Hodgkin's disease, bone marrow transplants are usually just reserved for those patients who have relapsed after treatment. The type of transplant is almost always an autologous one. The preparative regimen may or may not include total-body irradiation depending on the patient's previous history of radiation therapy. BMT has shown promise in the treatment of lymphoma, although the follow-up time for the study of BMT's effectiveness in providing long-term cure has not been nearly as long as that for the acute leukemias.

A more recent use of BMT has been in the treatment of advanced solid-tumor cancers. One of the most frequently used and high profile of those currently under investigation is autologous BMT for metastatic breast cancer. This is very likely due to the fact that breast cancer is one of the most common malignancies among women in this country.

Many times women detect their own cancer in the form of a hard, nontender, perhaps irregularly shaped lump in their breast when performing breast self-examination. Because even the very smallest lumps that can be felt may already contain a billion or more cancer cells, mammography (breast X-ray screening) is a very important, additional tool in the early detection of this disease. Changes in the breast and/or nipple, lumps felt under the arm, or even bone pain (from metastatic tumors) may be additional symptoms detected by the patient. Although it is rare, breast cancer can also occur in men.

Treatment for breast cancer generally consists of the surgical removal of the lump (a lumpectomy) or removal of most of all of the breast (a mastectomy). It may also include the removal of surrounding nodes and tissue. In addition, radiation therapy, hormonal therapy, and/or chemotherapy may be utilized. Chemotherapy is often given over a 6-month time period following surgery as an added treatment to hopefully kill any undetected cancer cells that could still be present and cause a recurrence.

Patients diagnosed in the later stages (Stages III or IV) or those who have recurrent metastatic disease may be candidates for autologous BMT. Peripheral stem cell harvesting, particularly for those who have metastatic disease in their bone marrow, may accompany bone marrow harvesting or be used exclusively to "reseed" marrow after aggressive, high-dose chemotherapy. Colony-stimulating factors are also commonly given at many centers to breast cancer patients after BMT to hasten the recovery of white blood cells.

Some of the other solid-tumor cancers that bone marrow transplantation has been used to treat are ovarian cancer, testicular cancer, some kinds of lung cancer, certain brain tumors (such as gliomas, one of the most common kinds of brain tumor in adults), and some kinds of sarcoma (cancers that arise in the underlying structures of bone or soft tissues). As in breast cancer, BMT is usually only reserved for cases in which a patient does not achieve or remain in remission.

Because BMT is used infrequently for these cancers, particularly when compared to the diseases previously reviewed, I am merely mentioning them and will not elaborate on each of them individually. (Refer to the sources listed in the appendix to obtain more information about these cancers.) When BMT is used, the type of transplant for these solid-tumor cancers is almost always an autologous one, done primarily as a rescue procedure to replace marrow destroyed by the high-dose anticancer therapy. Check with your physician, and the National Cancer Institute (NCI), to obtain more information about current clinical trials that are utilizing BMT in the treatment of solid-tumor cancers.

Childhood Cancer and BMT

Life-threatening illness is difficult enough to deal with as an adult, but it is perhaps even more shocking and unfair when it affects one who has barely begun to experience life. Although childhood cancer is uncommon, according to the American Cancer Society's *Cancer Facts & Figures—1993*, "cancer is the chief cause of death by disease in children between the ages of 1 and 14." In spite of this statistic, certain types of childhood cancer do have very high rates of remission and cure today. For those children who have a poor prognosis with conventional treatment, however, aggressive therapy followed by BMT can sometimes eradicate the cancer and improve a child's chances for long-term survival.

Cancer itself differs in many respects when it occurs in children. Adults more frequently develop cancers called carcinomas (which develop in the glands or tissues that line organs), whereas children more frequently develop sarcomas (which develop in bones, muscles, and tissues that support and connect other tissues). Differing patient size, maturity of body organs, cancer growth patterns, and tumor responses to treatment also make childhood cancers dissimilar to those of adults in many ways. Cancer treatments, including those used prior to BMT, are not only altered to reflect a child's smaller size but may also be adjusted to accommodate the differences in metabolism that can affect the absorption and clearance rate of medications. There are differing psychological and behavioral issues that also must be taken into consideration when the patient is a child. It is for these reasons that children with cancer should be treated at centers that have a team of medical experts who are experienced in pediatric oncology.

Some of the places in the body where cancer is more apt to originate in children are the blood, bone marrow, and lymph nodes; the brain and nervous system; bone and soft tissues; and the kidneys. Leukemia is the most common kind of cancer in children, accounting for approximately one-third of all childhood cancer cases diagnosed annually. Although it is still the number-one disease killer of children, mortality has decreased over the years due to improvements in care and treatment. Strides have been made particularly in the treatment of acute lymphocytic leukemia (ALL) in children, the most common kind of childhood leukemia.

Leukemia is also the most common childhood cancer treated with BMT. Although the vast majority of children with acute leukemia do achieve an initial remission from their disease, some types of leukemia are more resistant to conventional treatment. For these patients, more intense therapy, such as that administered prior to BMT, is needed to induce remission. For others, already in remission, BMT can sometimes make the difference between eventual relapse and total cure. This is particularly true for children with acute myelogenous leukemia (AML). For children who develop chronic myelogenous leukemia (CML), allogeneic BMT presently offers the only real hope for cure.

Allogeneic BMT, using a related HLA-matched donor, is generally the preferred type of transplant for the acute leukemias as well. Unfortunately some children who need transplants just don't have an HLA-matched donor. For these patients, sometimes an autologous transplant or unrelated donor transplant (if found) can be performed instead.

Even when there is a related donor, the family faces some special concerns when a child needs a donor for the transplant. Since those who are most likely to be HLA matches are siblings, the donor will probably be one of the child's brothers or sisters (who is usually also a child). Although the bone marrow donation process is generally considered to be a safe one, parents must confront ethical questions when agreeing to submit a healthy child to a procedure that is not medically necessary for him or her, particularly if the child is extremely young. This is generally not an issue for most of the other childhood cancers treated with BMT, because the transplant type is usually an autologous one.

Brain tumors are the second most common kind of cancer found in children. They may be difficult to diagnose, because sometimes their symptoms can mimic those of other less serious conditions. These symptoms include some or all of the following: recurrent headaches (which may be worse upon awakening), nausea, vomiting, sluggishness, drowsiness, speech disturbances, visual problems (such as blurred or double vision), seizures, and coordination problems that tend to worsen with time. This includes problems walking and maintaining balance, and difficulties in handling items and performing tasks. Brain tumors may be treated with surgery, radiation therapy, and/or chemotherapy depending upon the kind of tumor and where it is located. Although brain cancer is included in the list of those for which BMT has been used, it is an uncommon treatment.

Clinical trials (programs in which new treatments are investigated) utilizing BMT may be found at some oncology research centers for select kinds of tumors.

Other types of cancer that might necessitate the use of BMT in children are Hodgkin's disease, non-Hodgkin's lymphoma, and a number of other malignancies that predominantly occur only in children, such as Ewing's sarcoma, rhabdomyosarcoma, neuroblastoma, retinoblastoma, and Wilms' tumor. The lymphomas have previously been discussed, however, there are a few points worthy of mention in regard to their significance in children. Although Hodgkin's disease is uncommon among very young children, one of its peak incidence times is during adolescence and young adulthood. Because this is also a peak time for children to exert their independence and forge a life for themselves outside of their families, there are a number of behavioral and psychological issues that can make this a particularly trying experience for the patients and their families. Sometimes problems in communication and lack of compliance in following medical advice are encountered when the patient is a teenager. Fortunately, dramatic improvements in treating Hodgkin's disease, particularly when diagnosed early, have made BMT unnecessary in the vast majority of cases.

Improved therapies for non-Hodgkin's lymphoma in children have brought about increases in survival and cure rates, also. The high-grade, more acute types of non-Hodgkin's lymphoma, such as Burkitt's lymphoma, are more common in children than in adults. Since the nervous system has been found to be one of the more common sites for recurrence of the cancer, children may be treated with preventative radiation therapy to this area. The high-grade lymphomas generally respond more readily to anticancer treatment than do the indolent, slower growing kinds more commonly found in adults. This is one reason why BMT for non-Hodgkin's lymphoma is needed less often in children.

Ewing's sarcoma is a type of bone cancer that rarely occurs after age 30. Its peak incidence is between 12 and 15 years of age. The most common sites of occurrence are in the leg and the area around the hip bone. Symptoms include pain and/or swelling at the site of the cancer. Even for localized disease that appears not to have spread, treatment may include surgery, radiation therapy, and chemotherapy because of its high probability of metastasizing (particularly to other bones, the bone marrow, and the lungs). Symptoms that may indicate more extensive disease are weight loss, fatigue, and fever. Because of this disease's highly malignant nature, BMT may be needed so that higher doses of anticancer treatment can be given.

Rhabdomyosarcoma, a cancer that originates in muscle tissue, is the most common soft tissue sarcoma found in children. It occurs most frequently in the head and neck or in the genital/urinary area, although it can also sometimes originate in the legs, arms, or other areas of the body. Testing often includes MRIs, CT scans, bone scans, and bone marrow aspiration and biopsy to determine the extent of the disease. Tumors are usually removed surgically and radiation therapy is used, if needed, to treat any remaining tumor cells. Chemotherapy is given to those with disease that has spread beyond the original site of the tumor and may also be given as a preventative measure even when no other cancer cells are detected after surgery. Children with disease that has metastasized or who have unfavorable types of tumors may be recommended to undergo more aggressive treatment, followed by autologous bone marrow transplantation.

Neuroblastoma is a cancer that occurs along the nerves that run from the base of the skull down into the pelvis. Symptoms may include a mass in the abdomen or neck; bone pain; weight loss; bruising or other abnormalities around the eye; irritability; and symptoms of paralysis, anemia, and/or bleeding if the disease is more extensive. It may be treated with surgery (to remove localized tumors), chemotherapy, and/or radiation therapy. Surgery may be the only treatment used in very young children (those under 12 months) because their disease sometimes diminishes on its own with time even if it has spread. Metastatic disease in older children, however, is difficult to cure, thus high-dose chemotherapy and total-body irradiation, followed by autologous BMT, has been used in some patients to try to improve survival.

Retinoblastoma is a cancer that originates in the retina (the thin layer of tissue lining the back of the eye). The retina's function is to focus light rays. This cancer occurs most often in very young children (usually under the age of 4) and is sometimes inherited. Symptoms can include poor vision, deviation of one or both eyes, squinting, and/or the appearance of a white spot where the dark pupil should be (caused by the reflection of the white tumor at the back of the eye). Children are evaluated by an opthalmologist (an eye doctor), and testing may include X rays, MRIs, ultrasounds, a bone marrow aspiration and biopsy, and a lumbar puncture (spinal tap). These tests are done to determine the size of the tumor and if it has spread to other body tissues, such as the bone marrow or the spinal fluid. Treatment is determined by the size and extent of the tumor, the presence or absence of vision, and whether one or both eyes are affected. The eye may be surgically removed or other treatments, such as radiation therapy, may be used to destroy cancer cells. Because the disease has not spread beyond the eye in most cases, the cure rate for this kind of cancer is very high. If the disease has metastasized, however, treatment with aggressive chemotherapy and sometimes autologous BMT may be used in an attempt to improve chances of survival.

Wilms' tumor is a relatively rare childhood cancer that originates in the kidney. This cancer occurs most often in children under 5 years of age. The most common symptom is a mass in the abdomen, although high blood pressure, pain, or bloody urine may also be present. It usually occurs in only one kidney, but can occasionally be present in both. Treatment usually includes surgery to remove the affected kidney and to explore the abdomen for any spread of the cancer. If both kidneys are affected, obviously both cannot be removed. If the disease has metastasized, it is most often to the lungs or liver. Chemotherapy is given to most patients, even if the cancer appears not to have spread. Radiation is generally used only for larger tumors or in areas of metastasis. This cancer has a relatively high rate of cure so BMT is only used in cases of extensive disease that have not adequately responded to conventional treatments.

Bone marrow transplantation is clearly a difficult treatment regimen for both children and adults. Deciding whether to proceed with a BMT is hard enough when you are making the decision for yourself, as an adult patient. It can be an even more complicated process in the case of children, when several individuals (sometimes with differing opinions) are involved in making the decision. The child's age, personality traits, and level of maturity all determine how involved he or she can be or wants to be in helping to make this tough decision.

As with all medical procedures that involve minors, parents must sign or cosign consent permits to give approval for treatment. This is done once the physician has thoroughly discussed the procedure and its potential side effects with the parents and child at the transplant center. A heavy burden is placed on parents when the ill child and a sibling donor are not old enough to legally give consent or participate in the decision-making process. This responsibility can feel even more overwhelming after hearing some of the frightening complications that can develop.

It is not unusual for parents to have feelings of anxiety, fear, helplessness, or guilt. Parents may even blame themselves for not detecting signs of their child's illness sooner or for being unable to protect their child from the rigors that accompany a life-threatening disease and its treatment. Some parents may find it helpful to talk to others whose children have been successfully treated with BMT (referrals may be found through the BMT center or other BMT support organizations mentioned in chapter 1).

Explanations about BMT must be specifically tailored to the cognitive level of the child. After information is given, it is extremely important to assess how well the child understands the information and what he or she is feeling, as well as to address any questions he or she may have. Young children may misinterpret data, and if they don't ask any questions it should not be assumed they understand all of what they were told. Although some of the information about BMT is very frightening, children need to know what to expect and why BMT is recommended for them. This is particularly true if they are old enough to be actively involved in helping decide whether to go ahead with this treatment. If a sibling is to serve as the marrow donor, counseling also takes place to ascertain that the child does not feel coerced, to explain what will be expected, and to reinforce that he or she is not responsible for the outcome.

Being honest with children, without overwhelming them with details, may help foster feelings of trust and increase cooperation. Even very young children are capable of understanding far more than many adults give them credit for. The key is to present information in an age-appropriate manner and to follow through by encouraging children to ask questions and talk about their feelings.

Truthfulness with the child's siblings and friends can also help to allay fears that cancer is something that can be "caught" from other people, or that this disease is the result of ill wishes or punishment for something the child has done. Siblings have many concerns and worries of their own, not just for their ill brother or sister, but for their parents and for themselves. They may feel such things as jealousy, anger, guilt, fear, confusion, and insecurity. They may worry about who will take care of them or feel ignored and abandoned (particularly if the place of treatment is far away from home and they are left in the care of others). Fostering an environment that is as warm, supportive, and nonjudgmental as possible may help them express their feelings, just as trying to maintain normal daily routines may lessen some of the turmoil in their lives.

Once the decision has been made to go ahead with a BMT, parents need to plan who will stay with the child at the place of treatment and who will stay at home, continuing to work and take care of any other children in the family. There are often no easy solutions, especially with the financial and employment pressures most families must deal with. The situation is further complicated if one of the child's siblings will be the bone marrow donor. This child needs a great deal of preparation and support, too. Try to arrange as many things ahead of time as you can (such as help with child care, transportation, meals, washing, cleaning, etc.), because many additional matters usually come up later on that need attention.

Although it is far from easy, parents need to try to do their best to take care of themselves, too. Sleeping and eating patterns are generally disrupted, and nutrition may be poor from grabbing fast food meals on the run. It is both physically and emotionally draining to spend hours sitting at the child's bedside and to repeatedly travel back and forth to the hospital. A parent's own health may suffer from the extreme stress and exhaustion that accompanies caring for and coping with a seriously ill child, in addition to dealing with the other day-to-day responsibilities. Setting aside occasional rest periods and private time are important to renew your energy and strength.

All of the cumulative pressures and stresses make this a time when marital difficulties may surface or intensify, particularly if problems existed before the child's illness. On the other hand, the experience can also serve to draw parents and other family members closer together. Keeping the lines of communication open is an essential part of preserving relationships. Because BMT is such a stressful experience, family members who are having a hard time coping should not be embarrassed to seek professional counseling at any time before, during, or after the BMT takes place.

Prior to admission, a tour of the transplant unit will be scheduled for the family and child. Becoming familiar with this environment and the equipment that will be used during treatment can help to alleviate fears. Visiting hours for parents are usually very liberal and may be unlimited and include overnight stays. Depending on the center, siblings under 12 years of age may or may not be allowed visiting privileges. This is largely dependent on the unit's infection control philosophies and policies.

Once the child is admitted, it is important for the "homebound" parent and/or siblings to maintain communication via the phone and correspondence, particularly if young siblings are not allowed entrance into the transplant unit. Pictures of absent family members can be placed in prominent places in the home. This can be done in the child's hospital room, too, if allowed. Check with the hospital where the transplant will be done to see if they have any recommendations or restrictions about what kinds of things may be brought along to the hospital. My center allowed a host of personal possessions. We were encouraged to have almost anything that made our rooms feel more homelike. I know pictures of my loved ones and other treasured items were quite comforting to me.

Maintaining normal routines (as much as is possible) and bringing along favorite toys and other items can help the hospitalized child feel more secure. During this time, it is often best to keep games, puzzles, and other activities relatively simple and easy to complete in a short period of time because limited concentration and fatigue are very common.

Coloring with crayons is one activity that is easy to do and the repetitive motions can be soothing for some children. Cassette tape players or radios for listening to favorite music or stories is another pleasurable distraction. My hospital had VCRs available for viewing recorded movies or shows. If you have access to this equipment, you might want to bring along favorite tapes from home. You might also want to rent or borrow a video camera (if you do not own one) to make tapes of family members, your home, or friends for the child to watch while he or she is away from home. Reading to children from books containing familiar childhood characters and stories can also be very comforting. You may even find computer or video game equipment available for older children and teens. Most centers have specialists who can help with providing educational and recreational instruction for children who are undergoing BMT.

Counselors and social workers are also available to help both children and their families through the BMT process. Children may experience a host of emotional reactions to the physical isolation, the invasive procedures, and the prolonged side effects of treatment. Behaviors can range from passive withdrawal to acting out in anger. Younger children are generally the most concerned about being separated from parents, bodily injury and pain, and having their movement restricted. Regression to earlier forms of behavior may be seen. Teens can have a particularly difficult time dealing with issues related to loss of control and dependency, separation from their friends, feeling different than others their age, changes in body image (such as baldness), and the probability of sterility after treatment.

There is no question that there are many valid concerns, from both an emotional and physical standpoint, to raise before a child is treated with BMT. Children, particularly those who are very young, have rapidly growing and developing body organs that may be more vulnerable to damage by high-dose chemotherapy and radiation. Future growth and development may be affected. It should be noted, however, that children are generally able to heal damaged tissue better and more rapidly than adults. This can lead to more rapid recoveries and higher rates of survival than experienced by adults. Because children tend to be more resilient, both physically and emotionally, when all things are considered, they may be more ideal candidates for BMT.

3

Making the Decision to Have a BMT

· ·

Anumber of factors must be taken into consideration by both the physician and patient before a BMT is recommended and accepted as the best treatment for a patient's cancer. This includes a careful evaluation of expected side effects and potential complications. Clearly, *your* own physician is the one to turn to with questions about whether BMT is a necessary or possible treatment for your cancer. Most often, physicians will discuss BMT with patients if they feel it should be considered.

Your doctor may mention BMT shortly after your diagnosis, as in my case, or after an inadequate response or relapse from initial therapies. Because statistically BMT can be more successful in curing some cancers when performed during a patient's first remission (such as in acute myelogenous leukemia), it may be discussed early. For other cancers, it is considered only after all other less toxic treatments have failed to eradicate the cancer. There are also some diseases for which BMT is presently regarded as the only potentially curative treatment option.

From the Physician's Standpoint

The kind of cancer a patient has is crucial in determining if BMT could possibly be of benefit. Obviously, the cancer must be sensitive to high-dose anticancer therapies for BMT to be curative. Unfortunately, some cancers remain very resistant to the treatments presently available, including those as toxic as the ones used prior to BMT. Not only is a patient's prognosis evaluated in terms of the particular kind of cancer and its predicted course, but also on the characteristics of his or her own cancer cells and the responsiveness it has shown after previous therapies.

The answers to the following questions are considered before BMT is recommended:

- How extensive is the patient's cancer, or tumor burden, at the time of diagnosis?
- If the patient has acute leukemia, is his or her white blood count extremely high (greater than 200,000)?
- Does it take 2 or 3 attempts to induce an initial remission?
- Does the patient have a cancer that tends to place him or her at high risk for relapse? Is an initial or lasting remission not attained from repeated therapies?
- Are there no other curative treatments presently available for the type or stage of cancer that a patient has?
- How have the patient's body organs (particularly the heart, lungs, and liver) tolerated previous anticancer treatments, and could they be expected to withstand the higher doses associated with BMT treatment?
- Does the patient have a slower growing, more chronic form of cancer that may still allow him or her many quality years without BMT?
- Is it worth trading this possibility for the risks associated with BMT?
- What is the patient's age at the time of diagnosis?
- How is the patient coping psychologically?
- And, most important, is the patient willing to undergo BMT if it is recommended?

Deciding if and *when* a patient should undergo a bone marrow transplant can be extremely difficult. If a patient is in remission, might he or she remain that way without undergoing a BMT? When I was treated, Dr. Santos told me that BMT should offer at least a 20% to 30% higher chance of cure or long-term remission than other available treatments to justify the risks involved. Consideration must also be given to any new protocols of treatment that have shown improved survival without using BMT. Just as advances are made in the field of BMT, they are also made in other areas as well.

If an allogeneic transplant is proposed, the critical factor to evaluate first is whether or not a closely matched, willing donor can be found. One of the first questions a patient is usually asked is whether or not they have any siblings, or other close relatives, available for HLA evaluation. If not, can a donor be found through a BMT registry, like the National Marrow Donor Program or the American Association of Bone Marrow Donor Registries? If no suitable donor can be found and an allogeneic transplant is the only kind considered of value to the patient, then unfortunately, BMT is no longer a treatment option.

Sometimes a physician may suggest testing family members just to ascertain whether an HLA match exists, even before a patient has completed his or her initial cancer treatments. This lets the patient and physician know if a related-donor match is available, if wanted or needed, for a future BMT. This was done in my case, and since I had a matched-sibling donor, my treatment plan called for me to undergo a BMT as quickly as possible after attaining an initial remission. My oncologist told me many times that I was an ideal candidate for an allogeneic BMT, not only because I had such a well-matched donor but because I was in a first remission, because it took two rounds of chemotherapy to induce this remission, and because I was at relatively high risk for relapse.

Autologous BMTs, however, are being used increasingly to treat acute leukemia in cases where the patient does not have a matched donor. As better ways of purging marrow of cancer cells are used, and particularly as new methods are utilized to stimulate the patient's body to destroy any remaining cancer cells after high-dose therapy, this type of transplant may become even more successful in bringing about a long-term cure. This would not only eliminate the problem of finding a matched donor, but would also remove the risks associated with the use of donor marrow.

If an autologous BMT is being considered for a patient who does not have a malignancy that originates in the marrow, some of the following questions are also evaluated to decide whether and how the BMT should be done:

- Are the tumor cells sensitive enough to high-dose anticancer therapies to make BMT a curative possibility?
- Has the cancer metastasized into the bone marrow?
- What, if any, marrow-purging techniques should be used?
- Should peripheral stem cell harvesting be used exclusively or in addition to marrow harvesting?
- When should the marrow or peripheral stem-cell harvesting be done?
- Should additional anticancer treatments be done first, to further reduce the patient's tumor burden prior to harvesting and BMT?

These and other questions are thoroughly evaluated as part of the decision-making process. The recommendation that a patient undergo BMT is never one that is made lightly. It is only advised by a physician after very careful evaluation of a patient's other treatment options, medical history, and current physical and mental status.

How a Patient Decides

You must take all the information your physician reviews with you about your disease into consideration when deciding whether to undergo a BMT. If you have an acute illness that is not responding to treatment and it is your only hope for a remission or cure, the decision might be a little easier to make, knowing that you may not live long without giving BMT a try. If you are in remission or have a chronic kind of cancer and still feel reasonably good, even if BMT is your only hope or best hope for a cure, it might be a little more difficult to decide if it is worth the risk or the right time for you to have a BMT.

Physicians make the most educated decisions they can, based on current medical knowledge, when recommending treatment, but ultimately only you can decide what's right for you after weighing all the facts you have learned about your disease and evaluating how you feel about undergoing BMT.

In spite of the fact that I was extremely scared to undergo BMT, I truly believed that it provided me with the best hope for a cure. I was not satisfied with only going for what could be a short-term reprieve from the cancer. Although I was fortunate to have the possibility of being cured from conventional chemotherapy, the odds of staying in remission were just not good enough to give me peace of mind. Therefore, I decided to trade the temporary "safety" of being in remission for the much higher initial risks associated with undergoing the transplant.

Not everyone feels the same way I did or is willing to do this. I know others who did not think BMT was worth the risk and opted for waiting to see what happened without it. Some of these patients are still doing well years later. But, of course, if you decide to undergo BMT and things don't go well, you may wish you had never done it, just as you may wish you had initially tried BMT if your cancer returns or intensifies. Unfortunately, there is no crystal ball that can tell what the right decision will be for you.

If you are contemplating whether to have a BMT, it is important to know that others have experienced very similar fears and uncertainties. It is a stressful and difficult decision to make. I often felt as if I was in a no-win situation. Neither having a BMT nor choosing not to have one seemed like a good idea. Although I chose to have a BMT, that's not to say there weren't times when I felt like backing out and not going through with it. Even now, years later, I sometimes wonder if I would have stayed in remission without undergoing a BMT.

You also need to decide if you're willing to accept a dramatic compromise in your quality of life until you, hopefully, achieve the good health you're seeking. The type of transplant, the intensity of the preparative regimen, and your age are all factors that can influence the duration of side effects and recovery time. You will be informed how long a BMT is expected to significantly detract from your quality of life before you agree to have the procedure. Remember, however, that recovery times are just estimates based on what others have experienced and do not specifically dictate how long your recovery will take.

Finally, consider how strong you are emotionally, because the journey ahead may be a long and arduous one. Evaluate how much help you will have getting through this difficult period in your life. Think about the resources you and your family have or will need to get through the stressful weeks and months before, during, and after your transplant. And once you do make the decision in favor of BMT, try not to be swayed or frightened by tales you may hear of others who experienced serious complications or did not survive BMT.

That's not to say you can't change your mind or postpone the procedure if you have second thoughts. But if you feel relatively sure that this is what you want to do, try to maintain as positive an outlook as you can muster. Find someone to talk to who has been through the BMT experience and is doing well, and focus on making plans in preparation for your transplant so you will be as prepared as you can be. If a related donor is involved, try to maintain open communication at all times with him or her about what will be expected of both of you during this procedure. Feeling confident that your donor feels committed to following through with his or her part in your treatment can greatly reassure you as you prepare for the BMT and, particularly, once you have begun the anticancer treatments that will destroy your own marrow.

Before you are accepted into a BMT protocol of treatment, you will be informed by a physician at the transplant center of the many side effects and potential complications that can accompany BMT. It is after this, and often in spite of this, that your final decision about whether to undergo a BMT is usually made.

Exploring Common Side Effects

A patient undergoing a BMT will surely experience many side effects. Some of these tend to be nearly universal for all patients regardless of their preparative regimen. Although they are referred to as "common side effects," which may suggest that these occurrences are not particularly serious, they are often very intense and distressing for BMT patients. Even seemingly ordinary side effects can be temporarily debilitating and torturous on a day-to-day basis. The best way I can describe the feeling to someone who has not been through BMT is to compare it to having the worst case of the flu you have ever had. However, with BMT, you don't feel better in a few days or a week because the symptoms of fatigue, nausea, vomiting, weakness, diarrhea, fever, and achiness continue for many weeks.

The type of preparative regimen, the source of the transplanted marrow, and the medications given post-transplant determine to a large extent how severe and/or prolonged these side effects will be. Of course, each patient's unique physiological and psychological makeup influences them as well. Although many advances and discoveries have aided in the care of BMT patients, the first few weeks, as well as the first few months, are extremely difficult for nearly all transplant patients and their families. There are concerns about marrow engraftment, fear of complications, and anxiety about whether the cancer has been eradicated. In a more immediate sense, it is also because of having to cope with the side effects of a treatment that so dramatically impinges on your quality of life.

Side effects are caused by the tissue damage, irritation, and inflammation that result from chemotherapy and/or total body irradiation. These anticancer therapies destroy not only cancerous cells but also normal body cells, particularly those that replace themselves quickly. Some of the body's more actively multiplying cells are those in the bone marrow, gastrointestinal tract, reproductive tract, skin, and hair follicles. When anticancer therapies are administered in extremely high doses, such as those given before bone marrow transplants, these toxic effects are magnified. Sometimes body organs can even be permanently damaged in the process.

Gastrointestinal (GI) symptoms are the most common side effect for virtually all of the preparative regimens. They are often found at the top of any list of chemotherapy side effects. These are also the ones that patients tend to complain about the most. Not only are they extremely unpleasant, but they detract from the ability to fulfill one of life's most basic functions—that of obtaining nutrition through eating. Loss of appetite is the rule rather than the exception for BMT patients, and most are on hyperalimentation (complete intravenous nutritional support) at one time or another during their hospitalization. You may also hear hyperalimentation referred to as total parental nutrition (TPN) or hyperal. Even if an adequate caloric intake can be maintained, patients can still lose weight and become malnourished because nutrients may not be absorbed, metabolized, and used as they should be by the intestinal tract (called malabsorption) due to the drugs and their side effects.

The GI system consists of the mouth, throat, esophagus (food pipe), stomach, intestines, and rectum. This continuous "tube" that runs through the body is lined with actively dividing cells. Inflammation and irritation can lead to the development of ulcerations and sores anywhere along the entire GI tract. Mucous membranes (the layers of tissue that line the body openings that are exposed to air), such as those of the mouth and throat, are frequently affected. Mucositis is the medical term given to the inflammation of these cells. Symptoms can range from mild discomfort to excruciating pain. Medications, such as narcotics, topical anesthetics, and special mouth rinses, are used to help relieve discomfort. Patients may experience hoarseness and have difficulty swallowing. In addition, some patients produce copious amounts of thick mucus that requires frequent suctioning. If this is the case, the patient is given a hand-held suction catheter to use as needed.

Because of the risk of developing mouth inflammation (stomatitis), mouth sores, and mouth infections, patients routinely gargle with antimicrobial oral solutions, such as Peridex. Antifungal agents (like nystatin) may also be used to treat or prevent fungal mouth infections. One of the most common of these infections is thrush (caused by a species of *Candida*). A patient with this infection generally notices little white patches on the inside mucous membranes of the mouth and/or throat with accompanying soreness. As you can well imagine, any of the above can make eating a difficult and painful process.

The mouth can also become very dry due to salivary gland disturbances. Cracks may develop on the lips or tongue. Mouth rinses, artificial saliva preparations, and/or lip balms (like petroleum jelly) may be used to moisten the mouth and help counter these side effects. In addition, changes in the senses of taste and smell may occur. This can temporarily make food taste very different or unappealing. The sense of smell is often heightened, and even subtle odors may become overpowering and disturbing. A metallic taste may be present in the mouth as well.

Of all the GI symptoms, nausea and vomiting are typically the most common and aggravating to BMT patients. Although stomach cells are irritated by chemotherapy drugs, it is the brain, not the stomach, that generally controls nausea and vomiting. This can occur either when gastrointestinal receptors are triggered and send signals to brain receptors via nerves, or when certain receptors in the brain are triggered by chemical substances in the blood.

To counteract nausea and vomiting, drugs called antiemetics are given (*emesis* is the medical term for vomiting and *anti* means against). There are several different classes of antiemetics. Those that work directly on the central nervous system are usually the most effective. Unfortunately, these drugs can have some profound side effects of their own. They can cause dizziness, shakiness, restlessness, extreme excitability, or severe drowsiness. Because the center in the brain that controls vomiting lies close in proximity to the center that controls the lungs and heart, drugs that suppress nausea and vomiting can sometimes cause respiratory and cardiac irregularities.

Even with the liberal administration of antiemetics, nausea and vomiting can be hard to completely control in BMT patients. It may be an ongoing problem for some patients. It certainly was for me. I even had the dubious honor of being dubbed "The Queen of Nausea" by one particular physician's assistant. The good news is that these side effects, even if quite severe, do resolve with time, although it can be difficult to keep your spirits up until they do.

One other GI symptom that is common is diarrhea. Frequent, loose bowel movements can be caused by the anticancer regimen used prior to the transplant and by other medications, such as antibiotics, administered during the hospitalization. When the actively dividing cells that line the intestines are destroyed, enzymes that digest food are greatly reduced. The food and liquid that are not absorbed by these enzymes, as they would be normally, are then passed through the bowels and eliminated in the form of diarrhea.

This bowel irritation can cause cramping, gas, and excessive mucous production. Taking antidiarrheal medications and avoiding certain foods that can aggravate diarrhea, such as milk products, may help. This is one of those symptoms, however, that must often just run its course (no pun intended) until healing occurs post-transplant.

Some preparative regimen drugs tend to cause diarrhea more than others. Busulfan is one of the main offenders.

Since chemotherapy causes actively dividing skin cells to shed, skin usually becomes very dry, thin, itchy, and sensitive. Skin cells all over the body are susceptible to injury and breakdown. Skin rashes are not uncommon, and patients may find that their "sweat glands" do not work properly for a short time. It is not only the preparative regimen, but other drugs (particularly antibiotics) that can cause or exacerbate some of these side effects as well. Skin may temporarily darken, particularly at the underarms and groin, as a result of certain kinds of chemotherapy drugs, like busulfan. Patients may also notice changes in the color or odor of their urine and/or bowel movements as a result of the different medications they are given.

Just as skin is harmed by anticancer therapies, so are hair and nails. Fingernails may develop dark lines and become very brittle and crack. My nails were even affected by the chemotherapy I received at home prior to going for my BMT. When I went to Johns Hopkins, one of the physicians I met soon after admission looked at my fingernails during an examination and said, "I see you've had three cycles of chemotherapy." He said this without looking at my medical record. His informal assessment was indeed correct! I had undergone two initial cycles of chemotherapy and one maintenance cycle. He pointed out that he had simply counted the three distinct, horizontal dark lines on my thumbnail.

All of the preparative regimens result in hair loss (alopecia). Total baldness is the rule rather than the exception when high-dose therapy is given. Patients temporarily lose not only the hair on their heads, but have thinning and/or loss of the hair on their legs, arms, underarms, groin, and face (including beards, mustaches, eyebrows, and eyelashes). Although it doesn't all just drop out overnight, hair loss tends to occur rather quickly for BMT patients due to the toxicity of the treatment.

Although hair loss is one of the least important side effects from a medical standpoint, it can be very difficult for some patients to deal with psychologically. It may leave them feeling self-conscious, vulnerable, ugly, or embarrassed. Hair loss may be particularly disturbing to teens. Most patients, however, have stubs of hair growing back within the first three months after their transplant, and return to a "socially acceptable" hair length in six months to a year. (However, this "new" hair may be a different color or texture.) Hair regrowth varies from patient to patient and may return more slowly to those who were already bald from previous therapy before their BMT. Although it is uncommon, there is also a small percentage of patients who have a thinner hair regrowth due to some permanent loss.

The destruction of bone marrow cells is, of course, a major side effect of the preparative regimen. For those who do not have cancer in their marrow, it is an unfortunate side effect. For most BMT patients, however, it is a primary objective of treatment. This includes those with bone marrow cancers, those receiving donor marrow (to lessen the chances of rejection), and those with cancer that has metastasized to the bone marrow from another site. The destruction of existing marrow also serves to open up space in the bones for the new transplanted marrow.

Many serious side effects result from eliminating all, or nearly all, of the patient's blood-making cells. Patients require close observation and supportive care throughout the first couple of weeks, which are crucial, until the new marrow engrafts and establishes adequate numbers of platelets, red cells, and white cells. The longer it takes for these blood counts to return, the longer the patient's period of extreme vulnerability to developing complications.

Low platelet levels affect the blood's ability to clot normally, so when counts get too low, platelet transfusions are given. Patients need to be very careful during this time to avoid cutting or injuring themselves. Just blowing the nose too hard can rupture tiny blood vessels and cause nose bleeds. Bleeding can also introduce infection into the bloodstream. Patients may bruise easily and notice petechiae (small red pinpoint dots) on their skin.

A reduction in red blood cells equates to fewer cells to carry oxygen to body tissues, so in addition to platelet transfusions, red blood cell transfusions are given. Symptoms of a low red blood count (anemia) can include fatigue, weakness, shortness of breath, paleness, a rapid heart rate, dizziness, and headache. Before red blood cells or platelets are given to BMT patients, they are irradiated (exposed to radiation) to lessen the chance that infectious agents will be passed on to the patient and to decrease the danger of initiating transfusion reactions. If the transplant is an allogeneic one, the marrow donor may serve as the source for some of these blood products.

Without the white blood cells of the immune system, patients are obviously vulnerable to a host of infections caused by bacteria, viruses, or fungi. These microorganisms are present in the environment around us and within our own bodies. Although some of these organisms are pathogenic (capable of causing disease), others that normally coexist with man may become opportunistic and cause infections in BMT patients. A healthy person's immune system can usually prevent or fight off these microorganisms before they become a serious threat.

Severe and sometimes even life-threatening infections are a constant concern. Infection can occur in virtually any body part or organ, although some sites are more commonly infected than others. The respiratory tract (especially the lungs), mouth, gastrointestinal tract, intravenous catheter site on the chest, and urinary tract are some of the areas that most commonly become infected.

Transplant centers may have "culture days," as Johns Hopkins does, when routine cultures of the throat, urine, and bowel movements are taken in an attempt to detect infections early so appropriate treatment can be initiated. Cultures are also taken when patients have symptoms that indicate infection is present. Virtually all patients receive antibiotics during their hospitalization either to prevent bacterial infection or in response to signs of infection. Some of the most common bacterial infections are those caused by species of *Pseudomonas* and *Escherichia coli* (E. coli).

Even with the use of preventative antibiotics, patients may run fevers. These can sometimes be "fevers of unknown origin," as they are called, for which the infective source causing the fever goes undetected. If fevers continue in spite of antibiotics, patients are often started on amphotericin B, an intravenous antifungal medication. Some of the most common fungal infections are caused by species of *Candida* and *Aspergillus*. Although numerous medications are available to fight infections, some fungal and viral infections remain difficult to eradicate.

In women, vaginal fungal infections are apt to occur, because antibiotics, which wipe out normal bacterial flora, are so frequently used. These infections are treated with medications such as Monistat 7 (miconazole nitrate) or Gyne-Lotrimin (clotrimazole).

Two viral infections that are not uncommon in BMT patients are Herpes simplex (more commonly referred to as "cold sores" or "fever blisters") and Herpes zoster caused by the varicella zoster virus (more commonly referred to as "shingles"). Both of these infections usually develop from viruses that were present in the patient's body prior to transplant. They were lying dormant until the patient's immune system, which had been holding them in check, became suppressed. Acyclovir is the antiviral drug commonly used to treat such infections. Parasitic infections may also occur. Two of the most common types are those caused by Toxoplasma parasites and *Pneumocystis carinii*.

Another extremely common side effect from BMT is infertility, with permanent sterility being the norm for those who receive total body irradiation (TBI) and/or high-dose combination (multidrug) chemotherapy pretransplant. The category of drugs that are particularly known to cause sterility are the alkylating agents. Some of these are cyclophosphamide (Cytoxan), busulfan, thiotepa, cisplatin, carboplatin, ifosfamide, nitrogen mustard, melphalan, and carmustine (BCNU). This is not to say that there have never been children conceived after these preparative regimens, just that for most BMT patients it is unlikely.

The return of ovarian or testicular function depends largely on the patient's age, gender, dose, and duration of treatment, and on the kind of anticancer regimen the patient receives. This includes which chemotheraputic drugs are given, what particular combinations are used, and whether TBI is included. Regardless of the preparative regimen used, however, most women over the age of 26 do develop ovarian failure and early menopause. Some of these women may have already become infertile or menopausal prior to their BMT, depending upon their history of previous cancer treatment. It is important to point out that infertility and sterility do not equate to loss of sexual function. Sexual desire and function return to normal for most patients as their stamina and well-being improve.

The type of preparative regimen administered is also an important indicator in predicting future growth and sexual development in children who have not yet undergone puberty. Side effects for those who receive TBI often include decreased growth rates, lack of the development of secondary sexual characteristics, and sterility. Conversely, studies have shown that when only high-dose Cytoxan was used pretransplant, normal growth and development generally occurred. Because combination chemotherapy is most often used today in the treatment of cancer, children may experience some of the same side effects as they do when treated with TBI. Children are followed very closely post-transplant in regard to these factors, and hormone supplementation with estrogen/progesterone for females or testosterone for males is initiated if needed to aid in their sexual development.

Because most transplant patients are relatively young—in the midst of their childbearing years or have not yet reached them—the issue of sterility is an important one. It is not uncommon for patients and their families to feel powerful emotions of shock, anger, sadness, and grief when learning of this BMT side effect. With the expectation of becoming sterile, some men choose to have sperm stored at a sperm bank prior to undergoing their BMT if previous treatments have not caused infertility or sterility.

Finally, there are some cognitive and psychological side effects that commonly occur in patients. Patients and their families need to be aware that temporary changes in thinking, behavior, or personality may occur during BMT and understand why they occur so they will not be unduly frightened. These disturbances can be caused by the preparative regimen and may be additionally influenced by other drugs the patient is receiving, changes in nutritional status, alterations in sleep patterns, physical exhaustion, and the tremendous emotional stress and pressure that this whole experience generates.

Mood swings, depression, excessive lethargy, crying, anger, hyperactivity, and inappropriate behavior may be seen. Patients may even exhibit confusion at times and have gaps in their memory about events that occurred during their transplant. Some drugs can contribute to this by exerting an amnesiac effect. At the very least, almost all patients have difficulties with concentration at some time during their hospitalization. For most patients, this equates to difficulty, or even the inability, to follow along when trying to watch TV, read, or converse.

Sometimes patients are very quiet and uncommunicative. This may be because trying to carry on a conversation just takes too much energy, that mouth or throat problems make talking painful, or that they are feeling depressed. Other patients may take on a light-hearted, joking manner in an effort to deny or detract from the seriousness of what they are going through. Even if bizarre behavior is observed, no matter how atypical for that patient, be aware that it generally lessens and resolves as treatment side effects wear off and the patient's health begins to stabilize.

This does not mean, however, that there cannot be some long-lasting effects or changes, either positive or negative, in a patient's behavior or personality as a result of all they have been through in their battle with life-threatening illness. How dramatically BMT affects the rest of an individual's life depends on many factors, but a significant one is whether or not they experience any severe or long-term physical complications.

Considering Potential Complications

A number of serious and potentially life-threatening complications can occur during and/or after the preparative regimen and BMT. Before you undergo a transplant, you will be made aware of each possible complication prior to signing a consent permit. Although it is easy to become overwhelmed by these many frightening possibilities, it is important to keep in mind that most of them occur in only a small percentage of patients.

Some of these complications are the result of temporary or permanent injury to body cells and organs caused by the toxicity of the preparative regimen. Others are the result of problems with the transplanted marrow itself. The body organ most at risk to irreversible damage is the bone marrow that must be replaced with harvested marrow after treatment. This marrow-cell destruction places the patient at risk for developing severe infections or excessive bleeding. Other organs that are particularly susceptible to injury are the liver, the lungs, and the heart. After the infusion of the transplanted marrow, additional complications, such as graft rejection, graft failure, or graft-versus-host disease (GVHD) may develop in some cases.

Without a doubt, infection is one of the greatest threats to patients within the first 4 weeks post-transplant. Until the marrow engrafts and white blood cell counts recover, the patient's body is defenseless against invading or existing organisms. Many infections in BMT patients do, in fact, come from organisms that are already present within their own body. Most of these infections can be successfully treated. A few, however, are highly resistant to available treatment and remain quite difficult to eradicate.

Perhaps the most feared of these infections is interstitial pneumonitis (IP), a severe form of pneumonia, usually caused by the cytomegalovirus (CMV), that often progresses to respiratory failure and death. Although some medications are available to combat this infection, such as gancyclovir (which inhibits the DNA synthesis of cytomegalovirus), this particular CMV infection has the potential to be a very serious complication. The risk of developing CMV infections is greater for those who are CMV positive prior to their transplant. (This means that blood tests show they have been exposed to this virus in the past.) Patients who are also at increased risk of developing CMV are those who are older, those who have allogeneic transplants, and those who develop GVHD.

If a patient is CMV negative, great attention must be given to the CMV status of potential marrow donors. CMV-positive marrow places this patient at great risk for developing CMV infections after the transplant. For this reason, CMV-negative donor matches are used for these patients whenever possible. All other blood products the patient receives must be carefully screened as well to try to eliminate any exposure to CMV. Although there are other infections that also have the potential to be life-threatening, interstitial pneumonia caused by the cytomegalovirus continues to be considered one of the most worrisome infections that can strike a BMT patient.

The threat of severe bleeding and hemorrhage is also at its greatest during the first 4 weeks. Platelet transfusions are given to try and keep the patient's platelet count high enough to prevent this complication. Sometimes, however, it is difficult to keep platelet counts at acceptable levels in a small percentage of patients. Even with adequate or good transfusion responses, platelet counts are still far below those that are normally found in a healthy person.

One bleeding problem that can result from the administration of certain chemotherapy drugs, such as Cytoxan, is hemorrhagic cystitis. This is an inflammation and irritation of the urinary bladder that can result in pain and/or bleeding with urination. After Cytoxan enters the body, it is converted into active metabolites (chemically changed products) by the liver. One of these active metabolite by-products is acrolein, which is thought to be the causative agent of hemorrhagic cystitis. It is excreted from the body through the kidneys in the urine. When it comes into contact (particularly prolonged contact) with bladder cells, and it can cause irritation and damage that can lead to bleeding. Ifosfamide is another drug that is particularly known for causing hemorrhagic cystitis.

For this reason, patients taking these types of chemotherapy are instructed to empty their bladders often (at least once every one to two hours), and large quantities of I.V. fluids usually accompany the administration of these drugs to try to keep the bladder flushed out. Some patients have difficulty urinating or are unable to urinate as often as is recommended. These patients may need diuretics (medications that cause urination) or may even need to have a urinary catheter inserted temporarily.

Although the majority of BMT patients show little or no significant organ damage in the long run, temporary and sometimes even permanent damage can threaten or prevent recovery. Damage to heart cells from high-dose therapy can lead to cardiac arrhythmias (heartbeat irregularities) or heart muscle damage (cardiomyopathy). Lung cell injury can result in pulmonary fibrosis (a scarring and stiffening of lung tissues). Neurological problems, such as numbness or tingling, particularly in the feet or hands (called peripheral neuropathy), can occur as a result of nerve cell damage. Seizures or tremors can also occur as a side effect from various medications. Patients are given anticonvulsants (drugs to prevent seizures) if they are going to be receiving medications that have the tendency to cause them. For example, Dilantin (a commonly used anticonvulsant) is usually administered to patients who are receiving busulfan (a potential seizure-causing drug).

Another major concern when extremely high doses of anticancer therapy are given is the potential for damage to liver blood vessels, cells, and ducts. The liver is the single largest organ in our body and is located in the right upper quadrant of the abdomen behind the ribs. (Most cancer patients are familiar with being asked to take a deep breath while their physician presses with his or her hand in this area to detect liver enlargement or abnormality.)

We cannot live without the liver because it performs so many vital bodily functions. The liver contains enzymes that break down or convert toxins to less harmful substances. It plays an important role in the breakdown and metabolism of medications. Kupffer cells in the liver digest worn-out red blood cells and foreign matter in the bloodstream, such as bacteria. Liver cells manufacture bile, which is stored in the gallbladder and emptied as needed into the intestines for the digestion and absorption of nutrients. The liver helps regulate blood sugar concentration by storing and releasing glucose, and it plays a role in protein and fat metabolism as well. The liver also manufactures substances that help to regulate how quickly blood clots. It synthesizes most of the body's plasma proteins, and it stores essential vitamins and minerals, such as A, D, E, K, B_{12}, iron, and copper.

Symptoms of liver damage and malfunction can include some or all of the following: elevated liver enzymes (SGPT, SGOT, and alkaline phosphatase); liver enlargement and tenderness; ascites (which is excessive fluid accumulation in the abdomen); weight gain; peripheral edema (which is swelling in the arms or legs); and elevated bilirubin levels in the bloodstream (which causes jaundice). Jaundice is the term used when body tissues absorb bile pigments and take on a yellowish hue. This is particularly noticeable in the skin and whites of the eyes. The skin may also become very itchy. Urine may turn orange and foamy in appearance, stools may appear white or clay-colored (due to a lack of bilirubin in the intestinal tract), and confusion may occur as toxins accumulate in the bloodstream.

One liver complication that can occur as a result of the preparative regimen is venocclusive disease (VOD). VOD (you may see this spelled "veno-occlusive disease" in some sources) is a potentially life-threatening disease that occurs when fibrous deposits cause the liver's blood vessels to become obstructed. This can lead to a backflow of blood from the liver, scarring of the liver's blood vessels, and symptoms of liver dysfunction. Doctors at Johns Hopkins presently regulate patients' doses of busulfan, one drug that can cause VOD, by monitoring their blood levels. Instead of just giving standard doses based on body size, as had been done in the past, individualized doses are now given in an attempt to decrease a patient's chance of developing severe VOD.

Liver disease can also occur as a result of viral, bacterial, or fungal infections. Many liver infections are caused by organisms that are already present in the patient's body. When the patient becomes immunosuppressed and normal body flora is wiped out by antibiotics, the situation is ripe for them to become active. In the past, it was not uncommon for some viral liver infections, such as hepatitis B or C, to be acquired by patients through the blood products they received. Fortunately, patients have less risk of being exposed to these viruses today as blood is now screened for these and other viruses.

Graft-versus-host disease (GVHD) is another complication that has the potential to cause liver damage. GVHD is a disease that can develop following an allogeneic bone marrow transplant. It occurs when donor (graft) lymphocytes attack patient (host) body tissues because they recognize them as foreign. Although severe GVHD is a dreaded and potentially fatal complication, a mild acute case can actually be beneficial. This is because an immune response against foreign tissue may include the destruction of any cancer cells that might not have been eliminated by the chemotherapy or TBI. This is why an allogeneic BMT is preferred over a syngeneic or autologous transplant for leukemia patients.

GVHD does not occur following an autologous transplant, although some researchers at Johns Hopkins have learned how to cause a mild and controllable form of GVHD in leukemia patients undergoing autologous transplants. This is being tested because of the potential antileukemic effect that GVHD appears to have. Although cancer cells are eliminated from the marrow prior to its return, these patients have a higher risk of relapse than those receiving donor marrow, because they do not have GVHD. If patients' immune systems can be mobilized with GVHD to destroy any cancer cells that might remain elsewhere in their bodies (that were not destroyed by the preparative regimen), their risk of relapse may possibly be reduced.

Naturally occurring GVHD from donor marrow is, unfortunately, not always as mild and easily controlled as the artificially induced GVHD. It has remained a troubling and sometimes serious complication following allogeneic BMTs. Even having a perfect 6-antigen sibling match does not guarantee that problems with GVHD will not develop. It remains difficult to predict with certainty which patients will develop GVHD. There must be some other significant factors, not yet known or understood, that can play a role in the development and severity of GVHD. Hopefully in the future, more advanced tests will be developed to predict with even greater accuracy the suitability of a recipient and donor match. It is known that the odds of developing GVHD are greater if the patient is older, if the donor and recipient are of opposite sexes, or if the donor is a woman who has had multiple pregnancies. (Pregnancy can make a woman's immune system more sensitized to foreign antigens.)

There are 2 different types of GVHD, acute and chronic. They are actually 2 different diseases with separate symptoms and times of onset. Patients may develop both, only 1, or neither kind of GVHD. It is even possible to have both at the same time. Quoted statistics may vary from source to source or from center to center as to how often each of these types occur. This is because centers sometimes have different ways of preparing donor marrow and treating patients to try to prevent its occurrence. Overall, the incidence of GVHD has lessened over time. This is due to better HLA matching and to newer drugs and techniques used to prevent or control it.

In spite of this, acute GVHD is still not that uncommon. Nearly half of all allogeneic patients develop this disease within the first 100 days post-transplant. The odds are, of course, higher for patients who have unrelated or less closely matched donors.

Chronic GVHD occurs in approximately one-third of all patients, with onset ranging anywhere from around 3 months to a little over a year post-transplant. (The average time of diagnosis is approximately 4 months.) It can occur progressively in patients who already have acute GVHD, or its onset may be delayed until after a case of acute GVHD has resolved. Chronic GVHD can even occur in patients who have had no previous acute GVHD. This is called de novo onset, and it generally has the best prognosis of the chronic types.

The severity and extent of acute or chronic GVHD can vary greatly from person to person. It can run the gamut from being so mild that it is barely noticeable to being so severe that it results in multiorgan destruction and death. Acute GVHD is given a number, ranging from 1 to 4, that denotes its grade (or stage). Grade 1 is the mildest, while Grade 4 signifies extensive GVHD. This number is assigned after a patient undergoes a thorough evaluation, which includes examining the patient's physical signs and symptoms as well as blood and other test results. The stage may be upgraded if GVHD does not respond adequately to treatment and progresses.

One test I was given to grade my acute GVHD was a skin biopsy (referred to as a "punch biopsy"). A small piece of skin was removed with a device similar to a paper-hole punch. It was examined under a microscope and used to diagnose and assign a grade to my GVHD. Fortunately, I had a relatively mild case (a Grade 2), which completely resolved with treatment.

The areas of the body that are most commonly affected by GVHD are the skin, the liver, and the gastrointestinal tract. Patients with acute GVHD often have reddened palms, soles of the feet, and/or ear lobes. This skin rash can be more severe and widespread, of course, in worse cases of GVHD. Skin may even appear sunburnt and may blister and peel. Diarrhea and symptoms of liver involvement, such as jaundice and abnormal liver tests, also commonly occur with acute GVHD. Acute GVHD often completely resolves with treatment, and symptoms may last a very short time (a few days or weeks). It can, however, directly merge into the onset of chronic GVHD or worsen and cause serious complications.

Mild chronic GVHD has a favorable prognosis with treatment. Even some cases of severe GVHD do eventually resolve, although it often takes a number of years for the disease to burn itself out. During this time, it may flare (increase in intensity) only to be followed by a period of quiescence (relative inactivity). One of the symptoms of chronic GVHD is darkened, dry, and taut skin (with the tendency to sometimes crack and bleed). The skin may also have hardened, crusty patches and may peel. Vision may be blurry, and the eyes may be very dry and feel gritty. The mouth may also be very dry. Acidic foods and toothpaste can cause an irritating, burning sensation in the mouth. These eye and mouth symptoms are due to GVHD's assault on lacrimal glands in the eye (which secrete tears) and on salivary glands in the mouth. Liver abnormalities, sinus problems, and respiratory infections are also quite common.

More extensive GVHD can result in hair loss, premature graying of the hair, and a loss or "ridging" of fingernails and toenails. Respiratory problems can include frequent bouts of pneumonia and bronchitis. A particularly serious lower airway disease called bronchiolitis obliterans may develop. Weight loss and joint contractures (stiff, contracted joints) can also occur. The battle against severe GVHD is a difficult one, and in spite of diligent treatment, death can sometimes result (most often from infection or from body organ failure).

Immunosuppressive medications are the mainstay of treatment for GVHD. Drugs such as cyclosporine, methotrexate, and prednisone (a steroid) are among those most commonly used. These drugs suppress the immune system of the transplanted marrow to hopefully stop the attack that is being launched against the patient's body. Allogeneic BMT patients are usually started on immunosuppressive drugs pretransplant in the hopes of averting severe GVHD. Unfortunately, these drugs have a number of serious side effects that must be carefully watched for and managed should they occur.

Immunosuppressants (because they suppress the immune system) can obviously increase a patient's risk of developing serious infections. Antibiotics are routinely given during hospitalization and an oral antibiotic, such as Bactrim or penicillin, is usually continued for months following BMT to try to ward off infections. The drug cyclosporine is known to cause high blood pressure and magnesium depletion, therefore most patients must take magnesium supplements and some must also take blood pressure medication. Cyclosporine is extremely toxic to the kidneys. Creatinine levels in the bloodstream generally go up because the kidneys are not able to clear creatinine (a by-product of energy metabolism) from the body in a normal fashion. Steroids can cause fluid retention, mood swings, drug-induced diabetes, muscle wasting and long-term complications, such as osteoporosis (bone loss/weakness) and cataract formation (a clouding over of the lens of the eye). Symptoms from steroids are largely dependent on the dose and duration of treatment.

More severe cases of GVHD may also be treated with medications such as thalidomide or ATG (anti-thymocyte globulin). Some patients even undergo something called psoralen and ultraviolet light (PUVA) therapy, which utilizes ultraviolet light to destroy T cells. To prevent or lessen the severity of GVHD, some centers use techniques (such as the use of monoclonal antibodies mentioned in chapter 2) to remove T cells from the donor's marrow before it is given to the patient. Although T-cell depletion can reduce a patient's chances of developing GVHD, it can also increase the incidence of relapse or graft rejection.

Despite the fact that not all cases of GVHD can be kept under control, many can be. Treatments to minimize and control GVHD have improved in the past two decades and will likely continue to do so in the future.

Some promising studies currently in progress are utilizing new T-cell depletion techniques, removing certain T cells thought to initiate GVHD (called CD8 cells) while sparing other T cells (called CD4 cells) that are thought to cause an antileukemic effect. This appears to not bring about the negative side effects sometimes caused by T cell depletion while, at the same time, decreasing the severity of GVHD. Another potential GVHD-reducing treatment being studied is the pretransplant administration of the drug thalidomide.

Finally, the complications of graft rejection, graft failure, and/or relapse can occur after a BMT. Graft rejection can be loosely considered the opposite of GVHD. Instead of the transplanted marrow rejecting the recipient's body, in this case, the recipient's body rejects the transplanted marrow. In some cases, marrow will appear to have engrafted and begun to come back only to stop functioning. (This is not always the result of graft rejection by the patient's cells, but may be due to other factors.) In allogeneic transplants, this can happen if not all of the recipient's immune cells were destroyed by the preparative regimen. These remaining cells may then fight and destroy the new marrow.

For patients with marrow cancers, if their own cells do take over and repopulate the marrow, this usually means that they will relapse with their disease. A strange situation can also occur if the marrow is neither totally won over by one immune system or the other. Both may coexist together with a certain percentage being donor marrow and a certain percentage being the patient's own original marrow. This type of situation usually sets the stage for eventual relapse as well, although not always.

To determine the origin of the cells that have grown back after BMT, marrow samples are taken by aspiration and studied after engraftment has occurred. If the donor and the recipient are of opposite sexes, it is much easier to determine whose cells are in the marrow. If the donor and the recipient are of the same sex and the HLA match is a close one, more complicated tests must be done because it is more difficult to distinguish between donor and recipient cells. Studies using cell enzyme or antigen determinations and/or DNA analysis must be used to verify the source of the engrafted cells.

Graft failure can occur if cells in the transplanted marrow are too few in number or are damaged by drugs, infection, or other substances. This can prevent them from engrafting or from increasing to numbers that are substantial enough to function normally. In an autologous transplant, if a patient's marrow is heavily treated with anticancer therapy before it is returned to him or her, it may take an abnormally long time for marrow to engraft. Or if too many cells are destroyed, the marrow may not engraft at all. It is even possible in an allogeneic transplant for neither the donor's cells nor the patient's cells to grow after the transplant, although it is rare.

Obviously, graft failure is a life-threatening situation and a second transplant (reinfusion of marrow) must be attempted if the patient is to have a chance for long-term survival. The source for this marrow may be "back-up" marrow that was taken from the patient and stored prior to the administration of the preparative regimen, or it may come from the same donor or a different one, depending on the circumstances involved.

Even in the absence of all of the previously mentioned complications, there is the chance that the cancer may not be totally eradicated by this treatment or that relapse will occur sometime after BMT. Fortunately, the odds of relapse are often much less for BMT patients than for those who have undergone more conventional treatments. If a relapse occurs a year or more after BMT, second transplants may be offered to some patients. In spite of the numerous risks that BMT treatment entails, it is important to know that many patients do successfully recover, are cured of their cancer, and go on to lead active, fulfilling lives.

Preparing for the
Transplant
· · · · · · · · · · · · · · · · ·

Once the decision is made in favor of BMT, many preparations are necessary prior to a patient's actual admission for the transplant. A potential treatment center (or centers) must be chosen and the required pre-admission tests must be completed. In addition to the physical evaluation, support systems and coping skills must also be assessed and plans need to be made to provide support for the patient and family members. This is a busy time filled with much anticipation and tension over what the coming months will hold.

How the Treatment Center Is Chosen

Your oncologist is usually the one who makes the first contact with a prospective BMT treatment center in regard to your need for a transplant, although a patient or family member will occasionally call centers directly to find out information about BMT programs. However, a physician's referral, along with the transfer of medical records, is the normal procedure. Your physician can tap into the latest research that is being conducted at various centers, evaluate which program or programs have admission criteria applicable to your cancer, and help facilitate your more rapid entry into a program as a potential candidate. This can be particularly helpful in finding programs for cancers that are treated less frequently with BMT and in expediting admission for a patient with acute illness who has active disease or who is at high risk for relapse.

There are many factors that influence which transplant center your physician recommends. The first, and perhaps the most important, is which centers have the most experience treating your particular kind of cancer. When undergoing a treatment as complex and potentially dangerous as a BMT, it makes sense to have it performed at a center with as much experience as possible.

The importance of a center's size and experience was expressly mentioned in an article I obtained from the International Bone Marrow Transplant Registry ("Increasing Utilization of Allogeneic Bone Marrow Transplantation: Results of the 1988–1990 Survey" by Mortimer M. Bortin, M.D., Mary M. Horowitz, M.D., and Alfred A. Rimm, Ph.D., *Annals of Internal Medicine,* 1992, 116:505–512.) This study not only cited information about BMT's increased use, but concluded that "the effect of center size on transplant outcome is an important issue." For example, when studying those who had allogeneic transplants for early leukemia, they found that "the probability of treatment-related mortality was higher among patients having transplantation at centers in which five or fewer transplants were done per year than among those having transplantation at larger centers." Although it was not addressed in the study, it is also vitally important that children be treated at centers that have experience treating pediatric patients.

Unfortunately, because this is a lengthy and expensive treatment, cost may also be a factor in determining if and where you can go for a BMT. Virtually all centers want either insurance verification of coverage or a certain percentage of the costs up-front before they will admit a patient or initiate treatment. Most of us are aware of the battles that have ensued over insurance coverage of this procedure, particularly for some of its more recent uses, such as in the treatment of some solid-tumor cancers. (See chapter 7.)

Another factor that may influence the referral is the location of the transplant center in relation to the patient's home. Although this is of lesser consideration from a medical standpoint, it is one that dramatically impacts the finances and plans a family must make when preparing for the transplant. Unfortunately, most patients and donors do not live near an experienced BMT center.

After careful consideration, your oncologist will discuss with you which center or centers he or she recommends and may ask for your preference if more than 1 choice exists (which it often does). I know patients who went for interviews at 2 or more centers and chose the program with the treatment plan and atmosphere that made them feel the most comfortable.

Regardless of the proximity of one transplant center to another, they often use varying preparative regimens and/or marrow preparation techniques. These are tremendously important factors to consider because they can affect the outcome of the procedure. If there are significant differences, you must weigh these variations in treatment procedure and, with your physician's help, determine which program appears to be the most potentially beneficial for you. This can be quite difficult and somewhat frustrating, however, particularly when evaluating new techniques, because sometimes there's just not enough data in existence to aid you in your decision.

Another relevant issue may be how easy it is to secure a bed at the various centers. Larger, more experienced centers generally have more beds in their transplant unit, but they usually have longer lists of patients waiting to be admitted into their programs. I remember being told by a nurse in the transplant coordinator's office at Johns Hopkins that they had a hundred or so people on their list at the time of my transplant. It is important for you to realize, however, that even if there are a large number of patients on a waiting list, it does not mean that all of them are ready for their transplant at the same time you are. I know that I was placed on the list at Johns Hopkins by my physician before I had even completed my initial chemotherapy treatment. This is usually done so that by the time you are ready, your situation will already be known and will have been evaluated by the transplant department.

It is also important to understand that patients are not accepted for transplantation strictly according to when they are placed on this list or when their physician made the initial contact. Patients with acute illnesses, who are either in remission and have a high risk of relapse or who could not achieve an initial remission from conventional therapies, are usually given a higher priority status on the waiting list. These patients tend to have a smaller window of opportunity for a successful outcome from treatment; therefore they are generally considered first when a bed becomes available.

This can be extremely difficult for those with more chronic illnesses, because sometimes they may have to wait longer to secure a bed. I know a young man with chronic myelogenous leukemia who was contacted with an admission date 3 separate times before finally being admitted. Postponements can also be caused by former transplant patients who need to be readmitted or by delays in expected patient discharges.

Finally, centers have differing criteria for accepting patients. Some are more particular than others in regard to the types of diseases and the health status of the patients they will consider for admission. Although some oncology centers have expanded the size of their transplant units or opened new transplant units since the time of my BMT in 1989, there may still be waiting lists at certain centers. The physicians at these centers continue to be faced with making tough decisions about which patients they will accept for treatment and when.

What Happens Prior to Admission?

After your physician has contacted the selected transplant center, your first communication with them is generally through their BMT coordinator's office. The necessary pretransplant procedures are reviewed, your questions are answered, and an interview is scheduled with one of their transplant physicians. In addition, a tour of the transplant unit is usually scheduled.

At the meeting with the BMT physician, the procedure and its risks are explained. You will also be informed if they would like you to participate in any research studies. Some studies directly affect your care, while others are designed to collect information that may make the procedure safer or more effective for those who have transplants in the future.

Many phone calls are generally made between the center, your physician's office, and you in the months preceding your transplant. Arrangements are made for the required preadmission tests. Your oncologist and/or the center will tell you which tests need to be completed as part of your initial evaluation. Depending on your type of cancer, these may include an array of blood tests (including kidney- and liver-function studies); bone marrow aspiration and biopsy; pulmonary function studies (to check airway and lung function); a lumbar puncture (to assess spinal fluid); and specific sonograms, scans, X rays, or imaging procedures. The results of these preliminary tests are usually sent to the center by your oncologist, although you may be asked to hand-carry some paperwork or slides when you go to the center for your interview.

Additional tests, sometimes even repeats of recently completed tests, are administered at the transplant center. These tests often include an EKG; a chest X ray; sinus X rays (to screen for infection); a heart scan (to evaluate how well your heart is functioning to pump blood); a complete history and physical; and what seems like a mountain of test tubes that are filled with blood for extensive lab studies. Other tests may also be performed at the center depending on their preadmission requirements for your particular cancer. All of these various tests are required to assess the extent of your cancer and determine if you have any signs of infection, whether any substantial damage to body organs from previous treatments has occurred, and if your condition is stable enough to reasonably predict that you will be able to withstand the rigors of BMT treatment.

These test results are generally considered acceptable (in terms of reflecting your current status) if they are administered within 1 month of your admission. Sometimes, however, the physicians at the transplant center recommend additional treatments be given before they will admit you for transplantation. This may be in response to new or more extensive areas of cancer that are found during the testing, or just as an additional treatment to maintain a remission. This obviously means a delay in your admission for the BMT and may require that all or most of these preadmission tests be repeated.

If you will be receiving donor marrow, the donor will be required to undergo evaluation and testing as well, although it is not nearly as extensive. The donor will have a history and physical, an EKG, a chest X ray, and many tubes of blood taken for various lab studies. The donation procedure is reviewed, pretransplant counseling is given, and questions the donor may have are answered.

Along with your initial interview and tour of the transplant unit, you may also be scheduled to meet with a social worker, who will give you information about the center's support services, the hospital, and the surrounding area. This usually includes suggestions concerning where family members can stay, where parking facilities are located, what public and hospital-related transportation is available, where restaurants and dining rooms are located, and other practical information that can be extremely helpful. If desired, you can request a packet containing this information ahead of time to aid in making plans.

Since families (and patients requiring outpatient care) usually reside in the center's area for many months, it may take a number of weeks for a vacancy to occur at one of the local housing facilities. For this reason, patients and family members are encouraged to make a decision about housing and have their names added to a waiting list as soon as possible prior to the transplant.

Cost is also an important factor for most families to consider when choosing a place to stay. Most of the larger centers have residences, apartments, and/or hotel accommodations available at discounted rates for transplant patients and families. Depending on the facility, payment may be assessed on a sliding fee scale based on income. However, this can still be quite expensive even if costs are reduced.

One alternative may be to stay at an American Cancer Society residence, called a Hope Lodge. These residences are located near many of the larger oncology centers. They generally have no set fees, but instead accept donations based on what each family wishes to contribute. Each of these facilities provides a homelike, supportive environment for cancer patients and their families. Transportation services, on-site laundry facilities, housekeeping services, and linens are usually provided. Presently, there are approximately two dozen existing lodges nationwide. Each relies on local volunteers and the surrounding community for its support.

If the patient is a child or diagnosed when a child, another option for housing may be a Ronald McDonald House. There are 124 such houses nationwide, ranging in size from 4 to 84 rooms, depending on the location. Fees generally range from $5 to $20 per day, but there is no charge if a family is unable to pay. Each house is supported by their local community and by McDonald's owners/operators. As in most nonprofit organizations, Ronald McDonald Children's Charities are supported through the efforts of numerous volunteers. To find out if there is a Ronald McDonald House or a Hope Lodge near the center where you will be treated, you can contact the hospital's social services department or either of these organizations (see the appendix for more information).

Although it can be quite limited, some of the cancer-related organizations offer financial aid to help pay for travel expenses. One organization that provides substantial help with air travel is the Corporate Angel Network, Inc. (CAN). This nonprofit organization is designed to give cancer patients and a family member or attendant the use of available seats on corporate aircraft for travel within the United States. The patient must have medical authorization for the flight and require no special equipment or services en route. There are more than 350 members who have joined this network to provide this volunteer service to cancer patients. When using this service, transportation requests should be made as soon as definite dates for admission, discharge, or appointments are known (see the appendix for more information).

Depending on your particular situation, many other plans may need to be made during this time period. These practical considerations may seem mundane or annoying in light of the gravity of the situation, but they are nevertheless important in facilitating a smoother ride through the rough times that lie ahead.

Coping with Pretransplant Stress and Uncertainty

Since candidates for BMT have life-threatening diseases and are usually grasping at this procedure as their best or only hope for recovery, the wait for admission to a BMT center is often nerve-racking. It is extremely stressful when you don't know when, or even if, the transplant will take place. Particularly for those who like to make plans well in advance, not having a definite date for admission can create a great deal of anxiety. Due to a number of circumstances, sometimes patients only have a few days or weeks notice prior to their actual admission.

There are a number of other factors that contribute to pretransplant anxiety. Even with a tentative admission date, there is always the chance that something in your preliminary tests will disqualify you from meeting the program's admission requirements. Knowing that your future may hinge on the results can foster intense pressure. In addition, sometimes insurance problems develop or other postponements occur.

Patients may also be justifiably concerned about their physical status and worry about whether they have regained enough strength from previous treatments to be ready for their transplant. This can be particularly true for those with acute illnesses who are being sent for transplantation shortly after intense initial therapies. Patients may concentrate on trying to eat more nutritious foods, gain weight, or engage in strengthening exercises pretransplant to try and improve their cardiovascular and respiratory status.

It is not unusual to feel very nervous and more emotional than usual in the weeks preceding your transplant. This waiting period is typically a time of frequent highs and lows. Each phone call or correspondence from your oncologist's office, or the transplant center, may leave you feeling more encouraged or more rattled. Many patients are torn between just wanting to go get it over with immediately and wanting to delay it so as to have more time at home to prepare. Being accepted for admission often causes both relief and fear. For some, the longer they have to think about what is to come, the more heightened their anxiety becomes. They worry about the frightening aspects of the procedure and about the possible return or spread of their cancer while they are waiting.

Most patients reflect on how precious yet tenuous life can be. It is a time filled with both hope and anxiety about the future. Each day may feel as if it is moving by at an agonizingly slow pace. Or, it may feel as if the days are flying by too rapidly, and you are incapable of slowing them down. Although it is a time for savoring your family, children, and friends, it can also be a time when tensions arise in relationships from the stress and uncertainty.

There are added burdens due to the many plans that must be made. Patients and/or family members may need to organize bills, financial matters, and the household to make it easier for those family members remaining at home. Important papers, such as wills, living wills, and insurance policies, may also be reviewed. Young children may need to be enrolled in a day care center. Babysitters and/or housekeepers may need to be hired. Lists containing important information may need to be made. All of these important activities can contribute to both emotional and physical exhaustion for all involved.

Insomnia is a common occurrence for many patients and family members. Some people obtain short-term prescriptions for sleeping pills, or other medications, from their physicians or seek counseling if they are having a particularly difficult time managing the stress. It is often hard to concentrate on tasks at work or at home in the weeks preceding the transplant.

Relaxation techniques and diversionary activities can be extremely helpful during this waiting period. If you do find yourself feeling fairly well on a particular day, take advantage of it and enjoy yourself. Find fun things to do, activities that make you laugh and temporarily forget about what you are going through. But when you feel down in the dumps and want to spend some time alone, do so. If you want to talk, share your feelings with a supportive family member or friend. Stay attuned to the feelings of others around you, and their need to talk as well.

You may wish to join a cancer support group, read self-help books on coping with cancer, or find others who have already been through the transplantation experience to gain helpful tips and encouragement. Most BMT centers, and some BMT and cancer organizations, can refer you to a former patient who would be willing to talk with you. If you think of questions or have concerns about your upcoming transplant, don't hesitate to talk with your oncologist or someone at the transplant center.

There are a number of other things that might be helpful. Keep important phone numbers, addresses, insurance numbers, etc. in a prominent place for easy reference. Emotional stress can make it temporarily difficult to remember even very familiar information. Try your best to focus on the present, not wasting time worrying about what has happened in the past or what is about to come. Acknowledge the things in your life that you do have control over, and as hard as it may be, try to accept the fact that there are many things about your illness and life that are not within your control. Focus your energies instead on those things that you *can* do to help yourself. Be willing to accept help when you need it, and acknowledge that others often feel the need to help you. Give them tangible ways they can do so.

Make plans and set goals for tasks you want to accomplish each day. This will keep you active and help you feel useful. Don't make goals too large or unrealistic, though, or you may create more stress for yourself. Find activities that promote feelings of well-being. For example, if you are watching a particular news story, TV show, or movie that is upsetting or depressing, turn it off or walk away from it. I know there were times when my emotions were very close to the surface. I could not bear to watch news programs or intense dramatic shows and movies, because I could not deal with the violence, suffering, or inhumanity to others without feeling upset or crying.

The same can be true for reading material. I remember reading one self-help book that made me feel responsible for causing my illness, because I "just did not love myself enough." Not exactly what I needed to hear at the time! You may also want to avoid people who are pessimistic about your chances for survival and treat you as if you are doomed. I remember a few of the looks and expressions of pity I got and how demoralizing it was. Be sensitive to your needs in this regard, and don't label yourself as weak for avoiding people or things that you find upsetting.

Crying when you need the emotional release, instead of keeping your feelings bottled up inside, may help you feel better. You do not have to try to maintain a strong facade in front of others if you are feeling upset or depressed. Let's face it, having cancer stinks! If you have times of severe or prolonged distress, though, don't consider it a weakness or be too proud to accept professional counseling. It may help you get through a particularly tough time and give you some valuable coping tools to use in the future.

Above all, try to savor whatever joy you find in each day and focus on the positive as much as you can. Even in what seems like the worst of situations, there is almost always something that could be worse or someone who is in a worse situation. Give yourself pep talks from time to time to boost your morale. Other people have survived and have been cured, so tell yourself that you will be one of them. I tried to think of my BMT as the final treatment I would have to undergo in order to be cured and gave thanks that there was a treatment that had the potential to cure my cancer. In addition, I felt the satisfaction of knowing that I was doing everything that was humanly possible to eradicate my cancer.

5

What to Expect During Treatment

. . . .

You will be cared for in a protective environment by a team of medical professionals who are experienced in supporting patients through all phases of BMT treatment. Many routine procedures will be carried out as part of your ongoing care. In addition, you will be given recommendations for what you can do to facilitate your care and recovery during this time. Although it is a demanding treatment, both physically and psychologically, focusing on each stage of treatment step by step and on each sign of progress (no matter how small) may help keep the enormity of the procedure, its risks, and the recovery time from overwhelming you and your family. After your marrow has engrafted and you have met the required discharge criteria, you will be allowed to leave the hospital.

The Hospital Staff and Environment

Oncology centers where bone marrow transplants are performed are usually part of large teaching and research institutions. They are often located near or in big cities. Bone marrow transplant teams consist of many skilled professionals because BMT patients require a great deal of specialized, supportive care.

Patients and their families come into contact with several of these specialists each day. The physician who is ultimately in charge of your care is called the attending physician. He or she is one of a group of doctors who have extensive education and experience in the field of bone marrow transplantation. They are under the direction of a physician who serves as their department head. This physician is generally a distinguished expert in the BMT field.

The hospital usually has a number of other physicians who assist the attending physicians. The fellow is a physician who has received an endowment from the institution for advanced graduate study (a fellowship). The fellow who works with BMT patients is usually in the process of receiving training to become a specialist in the field of oncology. He or she answers to the attending physician and may be in charge of overseeing other physicians who are in training, such as residents, interns, or medical students. In many hospitals, these physicians serve a "rotation" in the BMT unit for a month or two. The attending physicians take turns serving on the transplant unit as well. When not assigned to caring for patients, they move on to other professional obligations within and beyond the institution, such as research, teaching, speaking engagements, etc.

Other personnel that are directly involved in the care of BMT patients are physician assistants (P.A.s), nurses, nursing assistants, social workers, physical and occupational therapists, respiratory therapists, nutritionists and dieticians, and phlebotomists (who draw blood for physician-ordered tests). There are a host of other specialists who may be called upon to see patients having particular problems, such as psychiatrists, psychologists, psychiatric nurse liasons, opthalmologists, and I.V. nurse specialists.

BMT patients tend to become the most familiar with the nursing staff (particularly with those who regularly care for them). Most BMT units have a primary care nursing system, which assigns 1 or 2 nurses to coordinate each patient's care. They take care of the patient whenever they are on duty and communicate regularly with other members of the BMT team. This type of nursing helps foster communication and trust, and promotes more uniform care and identification of patient problems.

When the attending physician makes his or her daily rounds, the number of people involved in a transplant patient's care becomes evident by the horde of other medical personnel usually accompanying him or her. Initially, this can be quite overwhelming and intimidating to patients and their families. It can also be reassuring, however, to know there are so many people carefully evaluating you each day.

The actual physical environment of the transplant unit varies among institutions, as do policies and procedures. All centers have private rooms for patients and follow some type of protective isolation techniques to help decrease a patient's risk of developing infections. This involves the utilization of good handwashing techniques, air flow and filtration systems, and may include the use of masks, gowns, and gloves by personnel and visitors.

A sign will be posted on a patient's door reminding visitors and staff of infection control precautions that are to be followed before and after entering a patient's room. Sinks are usually located near the entrance of the room for staff and visitors to wash their hands. Patients do not use this sink, but instead have their own sink and bathroom that others may not use.

Air flow systems filter circulating air to decrease airborne bacteria and other particulate matter. Face masks help minimize exposure to respiratory and airborne pathogens. These measures are of particular importance when patients are "aplasic" (when their white blood count is less than 1,000, and their neutrophil count is less than 500). Protective isolation measures are usually continued until counts rise above these levels.

The centers that follow the most strict isolation practices have physical barriers, such as plastic curtains, that wall off a patient from visitors. There may even be specialized gloves or other methods used to hand items in and out of this isolation "bubble." In addition, all items that comes into contact with a patient while in this type of protective isolation are generally sterilized. A type of air flow system called a laminar air flow unit may be utilized. In addition to filtering air of particles, it blows air along parallel flow lines at a uniform speed.

Other centers have rooms that look more like traditional hospital rooms. They are still private rooms, but they do not have barriers in place that separate patients from visitors and others. Masks and protective clothing may not be required, although strict adherence to proper handwashing techniques are always followed. Air flow and filtration systems are usually present in patients' rooms, although they may not necessarily be laminar air flow systems. Some centers have air flow and filtration systems present in hallways as well. You may be given a choice of which type of protective environment you prefer if more than one type of room is available.

Visiting regulations vary from center to center. Some have age restrictions and prohibit young children from visiting patients. This is done to decrease a patient's exposure to childhood infections and diseases. Since BMT patients can have serious infections, it also prevents children from being exposed to any infections that are present on the unit. In addition, it decreases noise and commotion. Visitors who have a cold, the flu, or other symptoms of infection are told not to enter the unit. Live plants and flowers are not allowed in patients' rooms because they may contain insects, fungi, and other organisms.

Visiting hours are often similar to those on other hospital units, commonly ranging from 11 a.m. to 8 p.m. Hours may be more liberal and include overnight stays for parents if the patient is a child. They may also be more restrictive, particularly if a patient is seriously ill and requires intensive care due to complications. It is helpful to be aware of the unit's visiting policy prior to admission, especially if you have young children and need to prepare them for separation from a parent or sibling. Even if there are policies prohibiting children on the transplant unit, arrangements can usually be made before and after the period of aplasia to visit on a nearby floor.

Regardless of the physical design of the transplant unit, a number of aspects about this environment can make it a psychologically difficult place to be. If you are allowed out of your room, you will be aware of other patients and their status. A walk down the hall of any BMT unit makes it quite apparent that very ill patients are present. You may see a few patients on ventilators or hear of others who have not survived. The equipment and/or monitors present in rooms and at the nurse's station remind you of the seriousness of the proce-dure and its potential complications. Although you can hardly avoid being affected by those around you, try to focus on your own situation and on those you see who are doing well. All in all, it tends to be an environment that patients and their families never forget.

Pretransplant Cancer Therapy

As you will recall, the anticancer therapy that is given prior to a bone marrow transplant is called the preparative regimen or conditioning regimen. Its purpose is to eliminate cancer cells and prepare the body for the introduction of the transplanted marrow by destroying existing marrow. This serves to open up space in the bones for the new marrow. Because the preparative regimen kills both diseased and healthy white blood and marrow cells, the patient's immune system is consequently suppressed. This is of vital importance in allogeneic transplants, because it helps prevent the possible rejection and destruction of donor marrow cells.

Preparative regimens consist of high-dose chemotherapy or both high-dose chemotherapy and total body irradiation (TBI). TBI may be included as part of a patient's protocol because of its ability to reach all body cells. It is able to penetrate certain sites, such as the central nervous system, that chemotherapy cannot as effectively reach. If chemotherapy is used alone, more than 1 drug is almost always given, because combination (multidrug) chemotherapy has been found to bring about better overall cure rates for most kinds of cancer.

Many different chemotherapy drugs are in use today. Those most commonly used as part of BMT preparative regimens are:

- busulfan
- carboplatin
- carmustine (BCNU)
- cisplatin
- cyclophosphamide (Cytoxan)
- cytarabine (ARA-C, cytosine arabinoside, Cytosar-U)
- etoposide (VP-16)
- ifosfamide
- melphalan (L-phenylalanine mustard)
- mitoxantrone
- mitomycin
- mechlorethamine HCL (nitrogen mustard)
- thiotepa

Your preparative regimen may include one or more of these, or it may include others not listed. Consult your physician or the Cancer Information Service of the National Cancer Institute (NCI) to learn more about the protocols of treatment that are presently being used for your cancer.

Since there is no ideal preparative regimen for all patients, or for all patients with the same disease, protocols vary from center to center and may even vary within the same institution. This is often because research studies are constantly in progress to compare different kinds of treatments or to try new ones.

Differences may also exist among centers solely because they prefer one protocol over another. This is illustrated by the fact that one prominent center has a long history of using total body irradiation (TBI) and Cytoxan (cyclophosphamide) as its mainstay of treatment for acute myelogenous leukemia (AML), while another prominent center has routinely used Cytoxan and busulfan as its primary treatment for this same disease. Patients with AML have been cured not only from these protocols but from others as well. As you can see by this example, although BMT has been used for some time as a treatment for leukemia, even this disease does not have a standard preparative regimen that all centers use.

Finally, the preparative regimen you receive may need to be altered to meet your own particular situation. For example, patients who are not in remission may have additional anticancer treatments included as part of their protocols, while other patients who have already received extensive radiation therapy in the past may have TBI eliminated from their preparative regimens. Differences in preparative regimens exist and will probably always exist, so don't be confused or surprised if you are presented with varying treatment options.

Preparative regimens are usually administered over a course of 3 to 10 days. It often begins within a few days of being admitted to the BMT center. Of course, the length of treatment depends on the type of anticancer therapy you are going to receive. Except for the drug busulfan, which only comes in pill form, all of the chemotherapy drugs are administered intravenously. If you do not already have a central venous catheter in your chest from prior treatment, one will be surgically inserted before the preparative regimen is started.

If total body irradiation (TBI) is part of your preparative regimen, your entire body will be exposed to gamma radiation. These high-energy X rays penetrate all cells of the body. Since TBI is almost always administered in fractionated doses (a percentage of the total amount desired), you will have a number of individual treatments, instead of just one single treatment. This is done to try to decrease the toxicity and resulting complications that can occur in normal body cells.

TBI is generally given once or twice a day (at least 6 to 8 hours apart) over a 2- to 4-day period. The total number of treatments often ranges from 4 to 6. Patients are told to remove all jewelry prior to treatment and not to use any lotions or other substances on the skin while they are undergoing treatments. Transportation to the radiation department is by stretcher, and patients are usually required to wear a facemask while in hospital corridors to help protect them from exposure to airborne microorganisms.

Medication is given prior to each treatment to reduce nausea and cause drowsiness. This helps patients remain still during the radiation therapy. Positioning devices to support the body may also be used to immobilize the patient and maintain proper alignment. Patients are in the treatment room by themselves after the therapists position them. One side of the body is generally treated at a time and clicking or whirring sounds from the machinery may be heard when it is in use. Lying still in the required position may be uncomfortable, but the treatment itself is not painful. Treatments vary in length and may range from 10 minutes to an hour.

Because it is natural to experience anxiety about both TBI and high-dose chemotherapy, don't hesitate to ask the BMT staff questions or voice your concerns. The expectation of side effects, such as nausea and vomiting, and the fear of developing complications from this treatment are legitimate worries prior to therapy. It is important to know, however, that there are many measures that can be used to ease the discomfort and pain that these regimens can cause. There are also medications and treatments that can combat complications, if they arise. Be assured that both your physical and emotional needs will be evaluated closely on a continuing basis to help you get through this difficult time.

The Day of the Transplant

One or two days separate the end of the preparative regimen and the bone marrow transplant. Bone marrow is "transplanted" by intravenous (I.V.) infusion, through a central venous catheter, into the patient's bloodstream. This is a much anticipated, yet stress-filled, event for patients and their families. It not only signals the end of the total body irradiation and/or chemotherapy treatments, but sets in motion the process of planting the "seeds" that are needed for recovery. The actual transplant itself can be rather anticlimactic, however, due to its similarity to a blood transfusion. Nevertheless, patients and family members often have some vivid memories of the events that transpired on this day.

The day of the transplant is referred to as Day Zero. Following the transplant, a patient's "age" is given in terms of the number of days or months from this date. Sometimes it is even called a second birthday, and is almost viewed as a rebirth. It certainly is like starting anew, at least from an immune standpoint, because previously acquired immunity to disease is generally lost.

Transplant day is a busy one for the medical personnel involved in your care. A number of procedures and precautions are taken before, during, and after the transplant to monitor your response to the marrow infusion. This is especially important for those who are receiving marrow from a donor because adverse reactions are more likely. Bone marrow is administered slowly, particularly at first, to watch for signs of hives, chills, fever, or chest pain. The length of time it takes for the marrow to infuse depends on the quantity of marrow that has to be given. Marrow can take 4 hours or longer to infuse. Special machinery, monitors, and medical equipment may be brought into the room. Family members may generally stay with the patient during this time.

Patients usually have an EKG (an electrocardiogram) and a respiratory breathing test before and after the transplant. The results are compared to be sure that the heart and lungs did not sustain damage during the infusion. Patients are also usually attached to a continuous EKG monitor during the transplant, and may continue to be monitored for approximately 24 hours afterward.

Other tests, such as a chest X ray or an arterial blood gas (ABG), may also be performed after the transplant. An ABG involves removing a very small sample of blood from a patient's artery (usually from the radial artery in the wrist). This test is done to measure the levels of different gases that are present in a patient's bloodstream to assess how well his or her respiratory system is working.

Because of the extra care and monitoring you will need, your primary care nurse, or another nurse you are familiar with, is usually assigned to care for only you, or a small number of patients, on the day of your transplant. This is so he or she can spend a great deal of time assessing and monitoring your reaction to the marrow transplant. Vital signs (temperature, pulse, respiration, and blood pressure) are taken frequently. BMT patients are generally considered to be receiving critical care on the day of their transplant and sometimes on the following day, too, because of the one-on-one nursing care they require. I mention this so you will not be surprised if a few days of "critical care" charges appear on your hospital bill.

If a relative serves as the marrow donor, the patient and his or her family will undoubtedly feel additional stress on the day of the transplant. Although the marrow donation procedure is generally considered to be safe, with few associated risks, it still involves a surgical procedure and anesthesia. Family members often find the day is spent traveling back and forth between the recipient's and donor's rooms to assess their status and to offer words of comfort and support. Related donors may wish to visit the patient as soon as the effects of the anesthesia have worn off.

Although the day of the transplant is stressful for all involved, it is also a tremendous relief when this phase of the procedure is completed without complications. Even though my memories from this day are somewhat sketchy, I can clearly recall what the bag of marrow looked like, how long it seemed to take to infuse, and how extremely reassuring it was to finally have my sister's marrow safely inside me.

Routine Procedures and Recommendations

A patient requires a great deal of supportive care and vigilant ongoing assessment following his or her bone marrow transplant. The first couple of weeks are crucial, because side effects from the preparative regimen linger and blood production remains at a standstill until the transplanted marrow engrafts. Consequently, transplant units have a number of routine procedures and recommendations that they expect patients and their families to follow. These are intended to help prevent complications and to facilitate the care given by the BMT team. Upon admission to the transplant unit, these policies will be reviewed so you know what to expect, and what is expected of you, during your hospitalization.

The most common routines are those that revolve around protecting you from infection during the time your immune system is compromised. Protective isolation policies require visitors to thoroughly wash their hands when first entering a patient's room. Facemasks, gowns, and gloves may also be recommended. Visiting in other patients' rooms is prohibited to avoid the possible transfer of germs.

The importance of cleanliness and proper hygiene is stressed to all BMT patients. Daily bathing is necessary to help reduce skin bacteria. You may be asked to use special products during or after your bath, such as bath oils, skin lotions, or antimicrobial solutions. Shampoo, deodorant, perfume, makeup, and other toiletries are usually prohibited due to the skin's sensitivity and dryness. Although razor blades are not allowed due to the risk of bleeding and infection, you may be given permission to use an electric razor. Because hair is usually lost rather quickly, razors are not really needed anyway, except perhaps to shorten or remove hair prior to the preparative regimen so it is less messy as it falls out.

Keeping your mouth clean, to reduce bacteria, is also important in helping to prevent infection. Mouth rinses and foam swabs are frequently used in place of a toothbrush, because they are more gentle on the teeth, tongue, and gums. Toothbrushes can cause abrasions that may lead to bleeding or infection. The inside of the mouth is inspected regularly by members of the BMT team for sores, cracks, bleeding, and signs of infection, so that appropriate treatment can be quickly initiated to minimize discomfort or complications.

Because diarrhea can promote skin breakdown in the rectal area, special care must also be given to this part of the body. Patients are taught not to rub or wipe forcefully after bowel movements, but instead to gently pat themselves clean. You may be instructed to use disposable wipes instead of toilet paper or asked to sit in a sitz bath (a plastic tub, usually about the size of a large bedpan, filled with warm water; it is used to promote cleanliness and healing in the pelvic and rectal areas).

Patients may be encouraged to dress in comfortable, loose-fitting street clothes during the day, as opposed to wearing hospital gowns. Wearing regular clothes during the day and changing into night clothes at bedtime may help you to better distinguish between night and day, which may induce you to sleep better at night and be more active during the day. Fleece-lined sweatpants and sweatshirts were recommended by my center. I was told that this type of clothing would probably be the most comfortable if graft-versus-host disease or other skin problems developed. It can also be advisable because body temperature-regulating mechanisms may be altered. A comfortable, well-fitting pair of shoes (such as sneakers) is also beneficial, particularly if you develop any tenderness or discomfort in your feet.

It is important to adhere to the activity guidelines you are given during your hospitalization. Although you must be careful not to engage in activities that could cause injury, getting out of bed at intervals and moving about during the day may help prevent the complications that can accompany prolonged bedrest, such as blood clots, pneumonia, skin breakdown, diminished muscle tone, and decreased strength. Doing things for yourself when you are able may also help lessen feelings of dependency. At my center, I was strongly encouraged to get out of bed when I felt well enough. As a matter of fact, I was asked to walk a minimum of 20 laps around the unit (roughly equivalent to one mile) each day, if possible. Although activity is beneficial, adequate rest is also extremely important in promoting physical healing and emotional well-being.

You may also be asked to perform "lung exercises" with an incentive spirometer. This is a hand-held apparatus with a mouthpiece attached that measures the volume of air you are able to inhale when doing deep breathing exercises. Taking deep breaths periodically throughout the day can help keep the lungs expanded and possibly prevent complications, such as pneumonia. A respiratory therapist usually assesses your breathing capacity on a regular basis. Simple breathing tests are also done to check for signs of airway or lung problems.

Because infection can occur around the central venous catheter in your chest, the dressing that covers this site is changed every day or two by your nurse. This allows the nurse to inspect the area for signs of redness, drainage, swelling, heat, or pain. To help protect the skin, a common practice used at Hopkins was to fasten the catheter's "tails" to a gauze "necklace" instead of taping them fast to the chest. This eliminates the possible skin irritation that can be caused by tape.

Blood samples are routinely drawn each morning from your I.V. catheter to check blood counts, chemistries, etc. Your physician may also order additional lab tests throughout the day as needed. You are usually given the results of your white, red, and platelet blood counts each day. Some centers encourage patients to keep these daily counts on a calendar so they can better track their progress. This can help patients feel more actively involved in their recovery and provides a tremendous morale boost when evidence of engraftment appears and counts increase.

If you have agreed to participate in research studies that require testing, these will also be done at periodic intervals to obtain the information that is needed. Patients who undergo allogeneic transplants are watched closely after engraftment for signs and symptoms of graft-versus-host disease and may have periodic skin biopsies as part of the detection and evaluation of this disease.

Your vital signs are taken at least every 4 hours. If fevers occur, which they commonly do when blood counts are low, you may be treated with Tylenol, I.V. antibiotics, and anti-inflammatory medications. If fevers become too high, you may be placed on a hypothermia blanket (a "cooling" blanket) to try to lower your body's temperature. Cultures of the urine, throat, stool, and blood are usually done to try to detect the microorganism responsible for your fever. If fevers continue in spite of antibiotics, you are usually started on amphotericin B, an intravenous antifungal medication.

Along with frequent vital-sign assessment, you are routinely weighed (often twice a day or more). A rapid increase in weight can indicate a buildup of fluid. This may necessitate cutting back on your fluid intake or the use of diuretic medications to promote urination. You are usually taught how to measure and record your fluid intake and output. It is important for patients to cooperate by recording and saving the fluids that go in and out of their bodies so that an accurate, ongoing record can be maintained. Intake consists of the liquids that are taken by mouth, as well as those that are infused intravenously. Your nurse will record the quantity of I.V. fluids you receive each day.

Output consists of urine, stool, and vomit. Patients must save these bodily fluids so their nurse can view the color, quantity, and consistency of the fluids that are being eliminated. Patients urinate into a plastic "hat" that fits on the commode. The collected urine is measured before the "hat" is emptied. Stool samples are collected in a similar manner using a separate hat. Patients are generally instructed to vomit into an emesis basin instead of into the sink or commode. While this is unpleasant, it is nevertheless important and becomes a part of your day-to-day routine during this time. Even in the absence of symptoms, routine cultures of the throat, urine, and stool are usually done at periodic intervals in an attempt to detect and treat infections early.

Food intake is also monitored closely. Patients may be asked to record the quantity of food that they eat each day to assist the dietician in calculating a daily calorie count. (One way this may be done is by saving the menu paper that comes with each meal and writing on it the quantity that was eaten of each item, such as 1/4, 1/2, all, none, etc.) If a patient's calorie count drops below the minimum required for their size, intravenous nutritional supplementation (hyperalimentation) is generally begun. This ensures proper nutrition until a patient is again able to inject enough food and fluids.

Although patients may request favorite foods from outside the hospital, regulations may prohibit family members and visitors from bringing in certain types of food or from bringing in food altogether. Usually, foods containing egg products and fresh fruits and vegetables are restricted because of the risk that they might contain microorganisms. Spicy and acidic foods are often discouraged as well, because they can cause burning and pain in the mouth (particularly if mouth sores are present). Cold or cool foods are the most appealing to many patients, and small but frequent meals are often tolerated the best. Snack carts may be available to provide patients with palatable treats between meals. (Popsicles were always one of my favorites.) If patients are permitted to keep snacks in their rooms, usually only nonperishable foods are allowed. Always check with the medical personnel in charge of your care before eating any food not provided by the hospital.

All of these necessary routines and procedures can be quite difficult to cope with, particularly if your hospitalization is a lengthy one. The many rules and recommendations that you must observe can make you feel powerless, childlike, or rebellious. The daily, close inspection of your body affords little privacy and can be embarrassing. The physical isolation that is imposed during your period of aplasia can make you feel emotionally isolated from the outside world as well. (This can be especially true for those who are separated from loved ones and are far away from home.) Even if you are not in an isolation "bubble" environment, the fear of germs may make you reluctant to touch or hug others and cause you to long for direct human contact.

Most patients find it comforting if arrangements are made for a family member or friend to be with them as much as possible during this trying time. It can be very reassuring to know that there is a loved one nearby who can help communicate your needs to the staff and speak up for you if you become too ill to do so for yourself. Because there are so many emotional factors involved in this kind of intensive treatment and care, patients (and families) are assessed on a regular basis to determine how well they are coping. Routine visits by social workers and counselors are generally part of the ongoing care that is provided.

Length of Stay and Preparing for Discharge

Four to eight weeks is often the estimate given for length of hospitalization. The length of your hospital stay ultimately depends on many different factors. The strength of the preparative regimen needed to combat your disease, the severity and length of your side effects, the type of transplant you undergo, the procedures (if any) used to treat the marrow, how well the transplanted marrow engrafts, whether you are given growth factors after your transplant, and whether you experience complications that require further treatment are all factors that influence how quickly you recover.

For instance, an autologous patient whose marrow is heavily treated with anticancer agents before it is returned to him or her may have a more prolonged period of aplasia. This can obviously lead to more time in the hospital. On the other hand, a patient who receives growth factors after the transplant may recover blood counts faster and get out of the hospital sooner. An allogeneic patient who is having problems with graft-versus-host disease may have his or her discharge delayed for further observation and regulation of immuno-suppressant therapy.

Although the procedures used to treat your cancer and marrow can significantly affect your recovery, your body's response to these treatments is the most important factor in determining when you will be well enough to leave the hospital. Generally, your neutrophil blood count must remain above 500 per cu. mm. before it will be considered safe to discontinue protective isolation and hospitaliza-tion. (Your neutrophil count is roughly about half of your total white blood count.) Prior to discharge, it is often a common practice for patients to undergo another bone marrow aspiration and/or biopsy. This is done so physicians can more thoroughly assess how the bone marrow is functioning.

Before you are discharged, and throughout your entire hospital-ization, the hospital staff will teach you a great deal. You need to know what to expect during recovery, what precautions must be taken to try to protect yourself from complications, and what side effects require immediate attention. Patients are usually given a dis-charge booklet, as well as other written instructions. All medications that must be taken after discharge will be reviewed thoroughly before you leave the hospital. This includes information about why the drug is needed, the dosage, when it should be taken, and the potential side effects. Medications and other needed medical supplies may be obtained from the outpatient clinic at the hospital or from a pharmacy.

Although some patients are able to have their central venous catheter removed before discharge, many patients still need this I.V. line for blood transfusions and other supportive care. It may also be left in place as a precautionary measure. If it is not removed, a patient is given supplies and instructions to help him or her care for the catheter. Practice sessions are conducted under a nurse's supervision. Patients change their own catheter dressings and heparin well caps, and administer heparin well flushes to demonstrate that they know the proper procedures and techniques.

Outpatient clinic phone numbers and off-hours phone numbers are provided so you can get in touch with a BMT physician in case of an emergency. If there is to be a period of outpatient care following hospitalization, the first clinic appointment is often made for you. If you are discharged directly to home, you are given instructions on when to see your oncologist for follow-up care. A discharge summary and packet of information are provided for your hometown oncologist. This helps your physician provide care in accordance with the center's recommendations.

Some centers have a special meal or celebration in recognition of a patient's discharge from the hospital. My husband and I were treated to a catered meal brought in from a nearby restaurant. We made our dinner selections in advance from the restaurant's menu. A dinner table, complete with candlelight, was set up in my hospital room. It was a very joyous and memorable way to say goodbye to what had been a most difficult ordeal.

The transition from inpatient to outpatient care or the discharge directly to home, although a happy occasion, can also be a fearful one. It can be very scary to leave the security of the hospital. After being under the watchful eye and close scrutiny of the BMT team on a 24-hour basis, don't be surprised if you feel some apprehension about being responsible for your own care.

Patients are usually advised to have someone stay with them for at least the first few weeks or months of post-transplant care. Not only is the emotional support of value, but it is often a physical necessity since most patients are still quite weak and sick. Periodic assistance may be needed in order to perform your daily activities. In addition, the presence of a family member or friend serves as a safety measure to assure that help will be present should complications arise that require immediate attention.

What Happens after Discharge from the Hospital?

B efore leaving the hospital, you will be taught what you need to know to safely care for yourself as your recovery continues. You will also be informed what you can expect throughout the recovery process. Whether you will be required to remain in the vicinity of the BMT center for outpatient care depends on the hospital protocol and your physical condition. When you are discharged to return home, information for your local oncologist will be provided to help him or her guide your care in accordance with the BMT center's recommendations.

Outpatient Treatment

Most patients require a period of outpatient care before they are discharged to home. Even though the first 4 to 8 weeks following the preparative regimen are considered to be the time when patients face their greatest risk of developing life-threatening complications, some serious problems can still occur after that, particularly within the first few months. Therefore, intensive follow-up care is needed to monitor patients closely for signs and symptoms that could indicate serious complications and to promptly treat any that do arise.

Careful, frequent evaluation is also needed because patients usually are still quite ill and often require supportive care (such as the administration of intermittent blood and platelet transfusions, medications, and I.V. fluids). Although these treatments could be done at a clinic or hospital near your home, they are normally done at the BMT center so you can continue to be monitored by medical personnel who are skilled in recognizing, diagnosing, and treating problems specific to bone marrow transplantation.

Because of the risks associated with receiving donor marrow, such as GVHD, most allogeneic bone marrow transplant recipients must stay near the BMT center for approximately 100 days following their transplant. For some individuals, this means that the outpatient phase of treatment is as long or longer than their inpatient stay. Immunosuppressant medications needed to prevent or treat GVHD must be closely regulated, and side effects from the immunosuppressant therapy itself may need to be managed (such as high blood pressure, kidney impairment, low magnesium levels, and infection). In the absence of complications, doses of immunosuppressants are gradually lessened, and a patient's response to these reductions must be carefully watched as well.

Close observation is also particularly important during the first 100 days because the potential for developing interstitial pneumonia peaks between 40 and 80 days post-transplant. Interstitial pneumonia is a life-threatening lung infection most commonly caused by the cytomegalovirus (CMV). Allogeneic patients, especially those with GVHD, are more at risk of developing interstitial pneumonia. Patients who are older at the time of their transplant also have an increased risk of developing CMV pneumonia and other serious complications. (This holds true for patients who have had either allogeneic or autologous bone marrow transplants.)

Autologous bone marrow transplant patients experience many of the same side effects during the first few months following the transplant as allogeneic transplant patients. They are also at risk for some of the same complications. Therefore autologous transplant recipients, especially those treated for blood or lymph cancers, may also be required to remain for a number of weeks of outpatient treatment (sometimes almost until the 100-day point as well). Patients having either type of transplant can suffer from continuing preparative-regimen side effects, such as nausea or vomiting, which may require supportive care in the outpatient clinic. Likewise, subnormal or fluctuating blood counts and an immature immune system place patients at risk for serious infection or bleeding problems. Liver enzymes also bear watching during this time period, as some degree of liver impairment, although usually just temporary, is not uncommon. Allogeneic transplant patients, particularly those with GVHD, tend to show liver abnormalities during this early recovery period. Close monitoring is also essential to verify that the preparative regimen (and the purging techniques, in the case of autologous transplant patients) did indeed completely eradicate the cancer.

Certain autologous transplant patients, such as breast cancer patients, are more commonly discharged directly from the hospital to home following their inpatient stay. These patients are generally not as heavily pretreated with marrow-toxic, anticancer agents prior to transplantation, and therefore may not have as high a risk for complications following their hospitalization. When growth factors are administered after the transplant and the marrow is infused primarily as a "rescue" procedure, instead of to treat a marrow or lymphatic cancer, patients can usually be just as safely supported by their hometown oncologist during recovery as they could be as an outpatient at the BMT center.

Patients who must remain at the BMT center for outpatient treatment usually move into the motel or housing facility where their family has been staying (unless they live in the nearby vicinity). If you are not within walking distance, or if you feel too ill to walk, transportation to and from the outpatient clinic is often available by hospital shuttle bus or some other form of public transportation. Most likely, your family will have already discovered the best transportation, laundry facilities, food establishments, and other services that you will require, thus eliminating your need to make a lot of immediate decisions and plans. This is extremely helpful because patients often are still coping with fatigue and other treatment side effects.

Most patients are seen in the clinic several times each week.

Some may need to be seen almost daily. Routine care is usually not given on weekends, although sometimes treatments such as blood transfusions may be provided. If you have a serious problem during evening or weekend hours, you will be able to contact a physician by calling the emergency phone number you received when you were discharged from the hospital.

Although procedures may vary somewhat from center to center, there will be similar routines that must be followed each time you come to the clinic. Upon arrival, after checking in at the outpatient registration area, usually your first stop is to have blood drawn for the various tests your physician ordered. This generally includes a complete blood count (CBC) and blood chemistry and electrolyte analysis. The lab technicians at BMT centers are usually quite skilled and knowledgeable in drawing blood from both central I.V. lines and from arm veins (if needed) because of their training and extensive experience with oncology patients. Central I.V. lines can be temperamental at times, and once in a while you may be asked to change position or lie down in order for blood to be removed from the catheter.

After you are finished in the outpatient lab, you will usually move to the clinic area to wait for your name to be called to go back for your examination. A particular primary nurse and/or physician's assistant may be assigned to follow you throughout your entire outpatient period. Whether you see an outpatient BMT attending physician at each visit depends on the center's policies and how well you are progressing in your recovery. I usually saw an attending physician only once a week. A physician's assistant handled my treatment and communicated with the physician about my care between visits. Regardless of who you see, you will have an in-depth physical exam and an assessment of any significant problems or changes in your condition. Additional blood studies, procedures, tests, medication changes, or the administration of blood products, I.V. fluids, or medications are ordered if necessary. Because of the frequent visits needed, patients quickly become quite familiar with this setting, the outpatient nurses, and other personnel who frequently participate in their care.

Some tests, such as throat, urine, and stool cultures, may be done routinely to screen for signs of infection. Other tests and procedures may be done based on how many days it has been since your transplant. This is often in accordance with the follow-up protocol for your disease or to gather information for research studies. Tests may include periodic X rays, scans, bone marrow aspirations/biopsies, lumbar punctures (spinal taps), and other procedures. If a patient had cancer in his or her central nervous system prior to the BMT, or has a high risk of relapse in this area, several chemotherapy treatments may be administered into the spinal canal as an additional follow-up therapy during the outpatient period.

Other members of the health care team that you may see regularly are pharmacists, physical therapists, and nutritionists. A pharmacy is usually located in or near the outpatient center. Along with the nurses, physicians, and other medical personnel, pharmacists can help answer some of your medication questions.

Some patients need continued physical therapy to regain lost strength and muscle mass. Therefore, they may be referred to the hospital's outpatient physical therapy department. Don't hesitate to take advantage of this service if you feel you need continued exercise therapy. It may significantly improve your stamina and contribute to a more positive outlook and increased feelings of well-being.

It is not uncommon to have problems maintaining an adequate food and fluid intake during this post-transplant period. Therefore, a dietician's counsel can be valuable. Often, a dietician will check in with you periodically at outpatient visits or will be available at your request. Following a BMT, an adequate intake of calories and protein to facilitate repair and growth of body tissues is important to aid in your recovery. However, this is often difficult to accomplish because of a decrease or loss of appetite along with the sometimes continuing problems of nausea and/or vomiting.

Dieticians can give you many ideas and recommendations about how to maximize the calorie count and nutritional value of what you are able to eat. Some of the suggestions I was given were to eat frequent, small meals; to drink beverages containing calories; and to add toppings, dressings, and margarine or butter to foods. These increases in sugar, fat, and calories are usually recommended just during the immediate outpatient period or for a couple of months following your BMT to restore your strength and nutritional status. They are not meant to be continued on a long-term basis and should be discontinued after healing has occurred and when appetite and weight return to normal.

Your intake of food and fluid will continue to be monitored closely during the outpatient period. It is not unusual for you to be questioned at each visit by your nurse and/or physician's assistant about how much you are eating and drinking. You may even be asked to record what you are eating and the quantity so that a calorie count can be estimated. If you are not drinking enough fluids, your urinary output may be decreased, your mouth and skin may be even drier than is common during this time, and changes may be noticed in your kidney function lab tests. If you are unable to increase your intake of fluids, you will probably be given intravenous fluids in the outpatient clinic. It is not at all unusual for patients to need this from time to time, particularly those who are having continued problems with nausea and vomiting, or for those who are receiving cyclosporine or other medications that can affect kidney function.

Throughout the outpatient period, you will probably be asked to keep a record of your temperature and any symptoms or changes in the way you feel. Patients are often asked to take their temperature at least 3 times a day (morning, afternoon, and evening) and more often if fever occurs. Any temperature over 38° degrees centigrade (100.4° fahrenheit) is one that patients are usually told to report. If this occurs, your physician will examine you and run tests to try to determine what is causing your fever. Before taking over-the-counter medications, patients must check with their physicians to be sure the particular medication is allowed and to confirm when it may be used. Products containing aspirin and ibuprofen are not usually allowed during the initial recovery period because they can interfere with the platelets' effectiveness in blood clotting.

Besides fever, there are a number of other signs and symptoms that should be reported to your nurse, physician's assistant, and/or physician. These include the following:

- difficulty or pain when breathing
- thick or discolored mucus production
- coughing
- shortness of breath or other respiratory changes
- chest pain
- dizziness

- heart palpitations or irregularities
- severe or recurrent headaches
- blurry vision or other visual changes
- excessive dryness of the eyes or mouth
- pain or stiffness in the neck
- difficulty walking or maintaining balance
- changes in the color, odor, or consistency of urine or stools
- difficulty or pain in urinating or moving the bowels
- nausea, vomiting, or diarrhea
- mouth sores or ulcers
- white patches in the mouth
- pain or difficulty swallowing
- skin changes (including rash, redness, swelling, bruising, soreness, or discoloration)
- pain or stiffness in the joints, muscles, back, or other body areas
- changes in the I.V. catheter site
- bleeding from any area of the body
- any other symptom that you find to be new, suspicious, or unusual for you.

Although it is an awesome task to remember and watch for the appearance of any of these signs or symptoms, it is very important to report any that do occur so that prompt assessment, intervention, and treatment (if necessary) can be initiated. Some symptoms can be an indication of a serious complication. Early recognition and appropriate therapy can sometimes minimize a complication and prevent it from becoming worse. Occasionally, it is even necessary for a patient to be readmitted to the hospital for treatment. Although this can be extremely disheartening, it is important to remember that temporary setbacks are not that uncommon and do not mean that you won't go on to recover without further difficulties after treatment.

It is not only your physical health that is of importance, but your psychological health as well. There will inevitably be a number of ups and downs along the way. If outpatient treatment is needed for an extended period of time, the routine of the sometimes lengthy outpatient visits can be extremely grueling and tedious. It's often a case of "hurry up and wait" as you go through each stage of the check-in, evaluation, and treatment process.

If you are having trouble coping or adjusting to the many changes that your body and mind have been through in the past few months, it is important that you let someone know. The responsibility of helping supervise your own care, of taking a number of medications according to schedule, of coping with continued or new side effects or complications from treatment, and of dealing with the fear of developing complications or of relapsing can become overwhelming for patients. Having so many rules and recommendations to follow can make you feel angry and powerless. Changes in appearance and body image can make you feel embarrassed, unattractive, and insecure. Being fatigued and ill a great deal of the time can lead to frustration and depression.

Remember that it is not a sign of weakness to ask for help. The stresses of this experience can easily cause difficulties for even the most well-adjusted people. Social workers, psychiatric liaison nurses, psychologists, and psychiatrists are all at the disposal of the BMT attending physician if a patient needs or wants these services. Many BMT centers have a support group for patients, family members, and friends. This can be helpful by providing the opportunity to share your feelings with others who are going through similar experiences.

Once you reach the end of your required number of outpatient days, and sometimes even earlier, you will be discharged to return home if your condition has stabilized and your marrow has shown adequate signs of recovery. Although some side effects and complications are not as likely to occur after the 100-day post-transplant point, you will still need to take very good care of yourself and be vigilant in noticing and reporting any signs or symptoms that could indicate or lead to a serious problem.

Recommended Guidelines During Recovery

A number of precautionary measures should be followed during recovery to help prevent complications. As always, it is important to follow the specific procedures and instructions that your treatment facility gives you. Although you may be observed closely at the BMT center as an outpatient for many weeks, your marrow still needs a great deal more time to recover fully. I was told that it takes approximately 1 year for the immune system to function normally. Obviously, you need to take precautions to guard against avoidable exposure to the infectious agents that are present in the environment during this time.

To help prevent breathing in airborne microorganisms, you may be told to wear a surgical facemask when indoors around others. Because you are accustomed to the normal microbes of your home and family, you usually do not need to wear a mask in your own home as long as you are around close family members. However, if a family member is ill, particularly if he or she is a young child (who will naturally be less careful or able to contain germs), you should probably exercise increased caution by wearing a mask until their symptoms have abated. Since germs are passed not only through the air, but are introduced into our bodies through hand-to-mouth (or hand-to-nose) contact after touching things in the environment, a facemask can help decrease exposure to germs by restricting access to these areas. At the very least, wearing a facemask can help serve as a physical symbol to remind you to be careful around potential sources of infection.

It is also important to question visitors and to forbid anyone who has a cold, the flu, or other transmittable illness from visiting you. In addition, you will probably be told to avoid coming into contact with anyone who has received the live (oral) polio immunization anytime within the last 30 days. Because BMT can destroy previous immunity to diseases, it is actually possible to develop polio if exposed to the live virus.

The same is true if you come into contact with anyone who has chickenpox, measles, or some other communicable, infectious disease. *If you are exposed to any of these diseases, contact your physician as soon as you are aware of the exposure.* In some cases, it may be recommended that you receive medication (such as the administration of varicella zoster immune globulin, which is given to those who have been exposed to the chickenpox virus) to ward off possible infection. Again, it is important to question visitors about these diseases before coming into contact with them.

Avoid large crowds of people, in which you are more apt to be exposed to pathogens. If you must go to crowded areas, such as the outpatient clinic or your hometown doctor's office, it is advisable to wear a facemask. If you need to make a trip to the grocery store or another public place, try to go when it is the least crowded. Particularly for patients on immunosuppressants, wearing a mask and taking antibiotics are generally recommended for about 6 months post-transplant.

Although facemasks do help screen out microorganisms and spores, they do not in any way guarantee freedom from infection. Therefore, a number of other important precautions should be followed in attempting to avoid infection. First and foremost, it is essential that you follow good handwashing techniques on a regular basis, particularly when you are away from home and in public places. This is even more important than wearing a facemask in preventing the transmission of microorganisms. Wash your hands before and after handling food and after using the bathroom. It is important to continue showering each day and to pay meticulous attention to proper hygiene. Avoid water that is too hot, however, because of its drying effect on the skin.

You should continue to maintain good mouth care as well. Once your blood counts have returned to more normal levels, you will be allowed to use a toothbrush again. Check with your doctor, however, before you resume using a toothbrush or dental floss. Rinsing with fluids or special solutions may be recommended to keep your mouth moist. The mouth often remains very dry for many months following BMT. Ask your doctor for recommendations if this is particularly bothersome to you. It is important to start seeing your dentist on a regular basis. Decreased saliva production can result in a greater incidence of cavities. Remember, however, to let your dentist know about your history of BMT because antibiotics may need to be administered before any dental procedures as a precaution against infection.

Skin generally remains very sensitive following BMT; therefore, you should take especially good care of it. Skin care routines that were followed in the hospital are often recommended to be continued for a time after discharge. Patients are usually told that it is all right to begin using some toiletries and cosmetics again, as long as they introduce only 1 new product at a time to verify that rash, redness, or itching does not occur. It is often recommended that you wait for a few days after trying a particular soap, deodorant, shampoo, cosmetic, etc. before trying another.

All BMT patients are advised to wear sunscreen when outdoors because the chemotherapy and radiation treatments leave the skin especially sensitive to the effects of ultraviolet light. Allogeneic transplant recipients must be extra careful. Some studies have shown that the sun's ultraviolet rays can worsen or even initiate GVHD. Therefore, it pays to exercise as much caution as you can to avoid excessive exposure to sunlight. Keep skin covered, wear a hat, and wear sunglasses to filter the ultraviolet light that reaches your eyes. It is important to remember that ultraviolet light is still present even on cloudy or hazy days. Sunscreens with a sun protection factor (SPF) of at least 15 are usually recommended. My center suggested using a sunscreen without PABA. PABA is an ingredient in some sunscreens that can cause reactions in certain people.

I was advised to take great care in protecting myself against sunburn for the entire first year post-transplant. After this time, sun exposure was allowed to be very gradually introduced and lengthened. I am still very careful, to this day, in regard to my exposure to prolonged sunlight. That doesn't mean, however, that I avoid outdoor activities. I golf, go to baseball games, and visit amusement parks, among other things, but I am careful to wear a hat and reapply sunscreen on a frequent basis when I am going to remain outside for an extended time. Although my transplant was several years ago, I feel that it is wise to continue to exercise caution, especially since my transplant was an allogeneic one.

Obviously, an activity such as swimming is not recommended until your chest I.V. catheter has been removed and the site has healed. When swimming, remember to reapply your sunscreen periodically because it does wash off. I was told to avoid swimming in lakes or public pools until after the first year post-transplant as another measure to prevent infection. A private pool or the ocean, however, is usually allowed.

Care should be taken to avoid coming into contact with substances that are toxic to bone marrow, such as gasoline, cleaning products, solvents, paint fumes, gardening fertilizers, and pesticides. I was told to be extremely careful with these types of substances during the first 6 months post-transplant. One of my physician's assistants told me that everyone should try to avoid exposure to these potentially toxic substances as much as possible anyway. Because I was told not to handle or breathe the fumes associated with cleaning products, it was suggested that I have someone else do the cleaning during this time if possible.

BMT recipients should also use precautions when it comes to exposure to animals, plants, and soil. This is because of their potential to harbor bacteria, fungi, or other organisms. During the first 100 days, exposure to all 3 is usually discouraged. After this time, it is generally considered safe to be around pets, plants, and to work in the garden. Cleaning up after pets (such as emptying cat litter boxes) and coming into contact with barnyard animals, however, should be avoided for about 6 months to a year post-transplant.

You will be encouraged to engage in appropriate physical activities during your recovery to increase stamina, rebuild muscle tone, and keep your lungs expanded. Walking, climbing stairs, and riding an exercise bike were all recommended to me. Since I was discharged from my transplant center in January, my husband and I purchased an exercise bike that I could use to continue my physical rehabilitation indoors at home. If you do wish to purchase an item like this, and it is recommended by your physician for use in physical therapy, ask your doctor for a prescription that confirms his or her order. Check if your insurance plan covers all or a portion of the item's cost. (When making the purchase, a doctor's prescription may also save you from paying sales tax.)

It will take some time to regain your strength and energy. Many factors, such as your age, previous physical condition, and the presence of treatment complications, influence how quickly you recover physically from your BMT. Try not to get frustrated if you don't bounce back as quickly as you expected. Activities should be gradually increased as they are tolerated.

Individuals recover at different rates, so don't compare your recovery to someone else's. Just as before your transplant, you may have more energy on one day than another. Take advantage of the days that you do feel well by engaging in some type of physical activity. If you remain rather sedentary for a period of time because you don't feel well, remember to continue to do deep breathing exercises to keep your lungs expanded and to change positions often until you feel well enough to move about again.

Estrogen and progesterone hormone replacement therapy may be recommended for some women who experience early menopause as a result of the preparative regimen. This is because of the post-menopausal risks of developing osteoporosis and/or heart disease. Treatment is often begun about 6 months following the transplant, after hormonal function has been evaluated. Occasionally, it may be started earlier if a woman is extremely symptomatic. However, hormone replacement therapy may not be recommended for some women post-transplant—such as for those who have had breast cancer. You will be advised by your doctor if hormonal replacement therapy is recommended for you.

It is not unusual for both men and women who were sexually active previously to initially have very little sexual drive after their transplant due to the side effects and rigors of treatment. A patient's energy level, post-transplant medications, feelings about appearance, relationship with his or her partner, skin problems (such as soreness or sensitivity in the vaginal or rectal areas), concern about germs and infection, and psychological status are all factors that can influence the return of sexual desire and function.

My center recommended that a patient's platelet count be 50,000 or higher before sexual intercourse is resumed. Obviously, good hygiene practices should be followed and until fertility is evaluated, birth control is initially suggested. For female patients who are experiencing menopausal symptoms, vaginal dryness may make intercourse uncomfortable or painful. The use of a water-soluble lubricating agent, such as K-Y Jelly, or a vaginal moisturizing product, like Replens or Gyne-Moistrin, may be recommended to ease discomfort. Sometimes estrogen-based vaginal creams, such as Estrace, may be prescribed. Men may experience temporary problems with impotence as a result of physical or psychological factors. Talk to your doctor if you have questions or are having any problems in resuming sexual relations.

If you still have your chest I.V. catheter in place, you will need to continue to care for it. The dressing and catheter flushes should be done using sterile technique to try and prevent infection or other complications. You should report any redness, swelling, discomfort, or drainage that is present at the catheter site. You should also report any fever, because this can sometimes indicate infection from your catheter as well.

If the catheter is not functioning properly or becomes dislodged, you must notify the clinic or your physician immediately. If the catheter dressing becomes wet, soiled, or displaced, it should be changed. As mentioned earlier, you will be taught how to take care of your catheter before you are discharged, if it is to remain in place. If you feel uncomfortable or have any questions about caring for your catheter, do not hesitate to ask for further instruction. Written instructions usually accompany discharge and should be referred to as needed. The catheter should not interfere with your ability to perform daily activities, but extremely vigorous activities that could pull, tear, or damage the catheter should be avoided.

It may take many months for your gastrointestinal tract to heal and function in a normal fashion. Therefore, it is important that you continue to follow the fluid intake and nutritional suggestions that you are given to the best of your ability. Don't hesitate to let the dietician at the clinic or your hometown physician know if you are having problems eating and drinking due to mouth sores, nausea, or vomiting, so that appropriate treatment and comfort measures can be initiated.

While your immune system is recovering, it is also important to take great care in handling food to prevent spoilage or contamination that could cause food poisoning. I was told to promptly refrigerate foods that need to be kept cold, to defrost frozen meats in the refrigerator instead of at room temperature, and to avoid eating foods that are undercooked (particularly eggs and meats). You may continue to be discouraged from eating fresh fruits and vegetables for a time until your immune system is more mature. When you resume eating fresh produce, foods should be washed thoroughly. It is also important to check with your physician before resuming the consumption of alcoholic beverages.

How soon you will feel ready and be given permission to return to school or work depends on a number of different factors. Although consideration must be given to each patient's situation, your transplant center may recommend that you do not return to work or school for approximately 1 year after your transplant. Patients who are doing well and who need to return to work for financial reasons, or who do not wish to remain off work this long, may be given their doctors' permission to return sooner.

Some post-BMT patients return to work or school on a part-time basis until they feel ready to resume full-time responsibilities. The type of work, presence of complications (such as GVHD), and susceptibility to infection, among other factors, are all carefully considered on an individual basis. Sometimes, arrangements can be made with employers for some work to be done at home. For children, arrangements for home tutoring can be made until they are well enough and given permission to return to school.

It is important for you to remember that you are a unique individual. You may recover more quickly than expected or at a slower rate. Take it one day at a time, and don't hesitate to seek prompt medical attention when not feeling well, especially during the first few months post-transplant. Recovery is usually a series of a few steps forward and one back. Try not to become too impatient. Take your medications as directed by your physician, and follow all recommended guidelines (no matter how inconvenient or annoying) closely. Your active cooperation and participation in your own care is essential and can even make the difference between life and death.

Follow-up Care

Once you are discharged from the transplant center to home, you will be under the care of your local oncologist again. A physician information and instruction booklet, results of your past and current lab work, and a discharge summary sheet (which reviews your clinical history, present status, and current medications) will be mailed to your doctor or given to you to deliver. This information provides your physician with guidelines for your care and apprises him or her of how your recovery is progressing.

Most patients are seen by their physician on a weekly basis for at least the first month after returning home. This is necessary to evaluate blood counts and perform frequent physical examinations. Medications are administered and regulated to manage continuing side effects, to help prevent complications, or to treat complications if they occur. If you had an allogeneic transplant, your examination will, of course, include an evaluation for symptoms of GVHD. Liver function blood tests, kidney function blood tests, and body weight are usually monitored closely during this time.

Because some patients continue to need platelet and/or blood transfusions after discharge, this must also be arranged. Blood products that are given to post-transplant patients are irradiated (subjected to radiation) to try to prevent the transmission of infectious agents. This is also done as an added measure to try to prevent GVHD complications in allogeneic patients. If a marrow donor who has a different blood type than the recipient was used, then type O blood is given until it has been firmly established that the recipient has converted to the donor's blood type. (Type O blood is the only type that does not have antibodies that react against other blood types.)

Once a patient's condition has stabilized, he or she is followed approximately every 2 weeks for the next few months. This often continues at least until the 6-month transplant anniversary. Some patients are asked to return to the BMT center for their first post-transplant checkup at this time. If you have not made previous arrangements with the center, someone from the bone marrow transplant coordinator's office will contact you to set up an appointment.

The disease for which you were treated and your type of transplant determine which tests and examinations are routinely scheduled at follow-up visits. If you are having any serious problems, additional evaluation may also be needed. Checkups may require a day or two to complete, because numerous blood tests, X rays, scans, respiratory studies, and a bone marrow aspiration/biopsy are usually necessary. You may have follow-up appointments with several different health care specialists.

It is generally after the 6-month anniversary that most allogeneic BMT patients, who are doing well, are taken off of immunosuppressant medications and no longer need to wear a surgical facemask when around crowds. Any medications that were taken to manage side effects caused by the immunosuppressants are gradually discontinued as well. This often includes high blood pressure medication, magnesium supplements, and antibiotics. The central venous catheter, if it has not already been removed, may also be taken out around this time. Having all of these protective measures stopped can make you feel a little vulnerable and scared at first but provides great reassurance and encouragement that you are well on the road to recovery.

The 6- to 12-month period after the transplant is usually a time when patients begin to feel better, both physically and emotionally. Most patients tend to resume more of their normal activities. As recovery progresses, patients tend to feel better about their appearance. Usually, hair has regrown enough to boost self-esteem, dietary concerns become less prevalent, and weight becomes more stable. Nausea, vomiting, and diarrhea have all generally subsided as a result of gastrointestinal tract healing and the withdrawal of immunosuppressants, antibiotics, and other GI-irritating medications. Strength and stamina will have also improved in most patients. Checkups with the oncologist at home may be extended to 3- and then 4-week intervals (depending on the patient's condition). Monthly checkups are often continued until the 1-year post-transplant anniversary, when a thorough follow-up evaluation at the transplant center usually takes place.

During the first year post-transplant, it is not unusual for shingles (caused by the varicella zoster virus) to develop, particularly in patients who are on immunosuppressants or who have low white blood cell counts. Shingles appear when this virus, which had been dormant in the body, reactivates. Initial exposure to the varicella virus usually occurs during childhood (with a bout of chicken pox). Reactivation of this virus tends to occur only when the immune system is suppressed (as it is post-transplant).

The virus spreads by way of nerves to the skin, where localized vesicles (blisterlike raised areas filled with fluid) erupt. These eruptions can cause intense itching, tenderness, and pain over the area of the affected nerve. It tends to run along a nerve pathway on one side of the body and most often involves the nerves in the chest. It can also occur on the face and follow along the nerve that leads to the opthalmic branch of the trigeminal nerve in the eye. This can result in impaired vision and eye damage. It is very important that prompt treatment be initiated to try and prevent the spread of this virus, particularly in immunosuppressed patients. Another goal of treatment is to prevent and/or manage the possible complications that can occur after shingles, such as nerve pain, wound infection, and scarring.

Because BMT patients are so susceptible to the spread of this virus, they are often hospitalized and given intravenous acyclovir (an antiviral drug). I was told that my risk of developing shingles within the first year post-transplant was between 40% and 50%, with the peak incidence occurring between 2 and 8 months following BMT. Not unexpectedly, I did develop shingles at 11 months post-transplant and was hospitalized one week for acyclovir treatment.

Reaching the 1-year post-transplant point is a real milestone, one that brings patients and family members great joy and relief. If there are no complications and no continuing immunosuppressant therapy, a patient may receive the first in a series of immunizations against disease at this time. (This basically consists of re-immunization with your "baby" shots.)

Pediatric doses of tetanus toxoid, diptheria toxoid, and an inactivated polio vaccine are often given. The pertussis part of the DPT vaccine that children receive is usually deleted. This is because it contains a live virus, and live-virus vaccines are generally avoided. A live measles vaccine, however, may be recommended by some centers for patients who are at least 2 years post-transplant.

Usually, vaccinations are not begun until patients reach their 1-year anniversary because of their body's general inability to develop antibodies to these immunizations prior to this time. Once it has been established (through blood tests) that a patient has responded to these initial vaccines, boosters are given at appropriate intervals as instructed by the center.

It is important to note that family members may also be asked to avoid vaccines containing live viruses, such as the DPT vaccine or oral polio vaccine. Patients need to discuss this with their physicians if they have young children or other family members who will be receiving vaccines, particularly if they are scheduled to be given during the patients' early recovery period.

Yearly detailed evaluations at the transplant center may be recommended for at least the first 5 years post-transplant. They are often scheduled around the transplant anniversary date. Many of the same tests are routinely repeated each year. If you develop any transplant-related complications between these regularly scheduled appointments, your physician may contact the center to confer with the BMT team. You may even be asked to go to the BMT center for evaluation and/or treatment if it is deemed necessary.

At the time of BMT follow-up appointments, some patients want to go up to the transplant unit to say hi to the nurses who cared for them during their treatment. I know I feel a special bond with those who took care for me during that time. It can be difficult emotionally, however, to return to the inpatient area. Don't feel there is something wrong with you or that you are weak if you feel upset by the sights and sounds of the BMT unit. It is normal to feel stress and emotional turmoil considering all you went through in this environment. If it is too difficult to visit, then don't and instead send a note or place a phone call if you wish to communicate with staff members. It can mean a great deal to staff members to hear from former patients who are doing well.

In addition to the recommended annual checkups at the BMT center, you will continue to see your oncologist at home on a regular basis for follow-up care. How often you are seen depends on how well you are doing and what guidelines of follow-up care are indicated for your disease.

Until 5 years post-transplant, I need to be followed every 3 months by my oncologist for a complete blood count (CBC) and a physical. After this time, appointments will be scheduled at intervals of approximately 6 months if all continues to go well. Annual checkups at the BMT center after 5 years may still be advised, although testing is generally not as extensive at these appointments. For example, I was told that I will not be asked to undergo an *annual* bone marrow aspiration at the center after I reach the 5-year mark.

Throughout the years that follow your BMT, you will continue to be observed at regular intervals by your physician for signs of late complications from treatment. Appropriate therapy, if indicated, will be initiated to manage any complications. Obviously, seeing your doctor for follow-up care as recommended and taking good care of yourself continue to be very important not only during your recovery period but for the rest of your life.

Post-transplant Issues

· · · · · · · · · · · ·

Obviously, the best possible long-term outcome from BMT would be that your disease is cured, and that overall you are healthy and happy. This is indeed possible! My own experience has shown this to be true, as has that of many other BMT survivors I have met. It is not only the physical and psychological aspects of this treatment that influence your life, but also the continuing insurance and financial concerns that must be handled. Some patients will, of course, have an easier time than others coping with these many post-transplant issues.

Physical Health

There is considerable variation among BMT survivors in physical, psychological, and social function following BMT. This was one of the conclusions drawn by M.A. Andrykowski and others[1] who studied 23 allogeneic marrow transplant patients treated at Kentucky Medical Center who were between 3 and 52 months post-BMT. Their findings indicated that while some patients had a complete (or nearly complete) recovery, others had significant problems. Not surprisingly, they found that older patients tended to report poorer functioning after BMT, particularly in the physical area.

Some of the continuing health effects that can occur in varying degrees are:

- fatigue
- decreased strength and stamina
- general pain or discomfort
- muscle cramps
- skin, joint, or eye problems
- lung, liver, kidney, or other body-organ dysfunction
- frequent infections
- sinusitis
- sleep disturbances
- memory problems
- difficulty concentrating
- sexual function difficulties

Some of these side effects are, however, more likely to affect those suffering from GVHD. Although some minor or moderate health problems are not all that unusual, most BMT survivors do report a good quality of life after recovery.

Just as there are complications that can occur during and immediately following BMT (see chapter 3), there are also late complications that can result from this treatment. A late complication is generally defined as one that continues or develops more than 100 days after the BMT takes place. Late physical complications can result from the transplanted marrow itself (as in the case of GVHD), from the chemotherapy and/or total body irradiation (TBI) that was used prior to the transplant, from a recurrence of the original cancer (a relapse), or from the development of a new type of cancer (called a secondary malignancy).

Unfortunately, GVHD can be an ongoing problem for some allogeneic patients. Although it is the chronic form of the disease that occurs around or after Day 100 post-BMT, patients can continue to experience both acute and chronic GVHD in the months and years that follow their transplant. In some cases, however, it does eventually burn itself out. Even so, patients may still be left with long-term side effects—such as skin, joint, respiratory tract, and eye problems— that negatively affect their quality of life. In a study by Syrjala and others[2] of 67 allogeneic BMT patients who received their transplants at the Fred Hutchinson Cancer Research Center in Seattle, GVHD was reported to be one of the important factors in predicting who would have physical-function difficulties at 1 year post-BMT.

The preparative regimen can also be responsible for the development of late complications. Although high-dose chemotherapy and TBI can cause initial injury to body tissues, it can also cause injury that may take some time to become apparent. Problems noted shortly after the transplant may continue and/or new difficulties may surface. The heart muscle can be irreversibly weakened, and the reproductive glands are often damaged, resulting in permanent sterility. Lung complications, such as fibrosis (a stiffening of lung tissues), can occur. When the lungs are less elastic, they have a reduced capability to expand.

Although most late complications are generally applicable to both adults and children, there are some special concerns in regard to children. In an article by Wiley and House[3], it was noted that "toxicities afflicting adults may impair a fully developed organ; (while) toxicities afflicting children can impede the growth of a developing organ. Although young tissues are more resilient after trauma, growth can be altered or impaired." As would be expected, total body irradiation (TBI) treatment can cause decreased growth and development in children.

Wiley and House also note that "of particular concern in the pediatric population is pituitary dysfunction, growth hormone deficiency, and other endocrine problems." (Endocrine glands in the body secrete hormones, which are chemical messengers. The glands that comprise the endocrine system are the pituitary, thyroid, parathyroids, pineal, thymus, adrenals, pancreas, ovaries, and testes.)

Neurological (nerve) problems can also occur after BMT. When radiation has been administered to the head or chemotherapy has been administered into the spine, something called leukoencephalopathy (damage to the white matter of the brain) can occur. Learning skills and memory can be impaired in some patients. Certain chemotherapy agents can cause peripheral neuropathy (numbness and tingling in the feet and/or hands). There have even been rare reports of patients developing myasthenia gravis as a late complication from BMT. Myasthenia gravis is a neurological disorder characterized by extreme muscle weakness.

Another possible late complication from BMT treatment is the development of cataracts. Cataracts, a clouding over of the eyes' lenses, can develop after total body irradiation (TBI) and/or steroid therapy. For those who received TBI, this may develop 3 to 6 years after treatment. The incidence is much less today, however, since irradiation is usually given in divided doses as opposed to one large dose (now there is approximately a 25% occurrence rate as compared to the 75% to 80% rate of occurrence in the past). For those who receive steroid therapy, the risk of developing cataracts is greater when steroids are taken for a prolonged period of time, particularly at higher doses. Steroid therapy also predisposes patients to developing bone destruction in the area of the hip, called osteonecrosis or aseptic necrosis of the hip.

Hearing impairment is another potential complication from treatment. It is usually mild, however, and more commonly affects high-frequency sounds. If hearing loss does occur after BMT, it is most likely the result of having received particular types of antibiotics (those from the aminoglycoside class). Examples of antibiotics in this category are gentamicin, streptomycin, and tobramycin.

Finally, a recurrence of the original cancer (a relapse) or the development of a new type of cancer (called a secondary malignancy) are other possible late complications following BMT. Secondary cancers are rare and are thought to result from past exposure to the irradiation, high-dose chemotherapy, or immunosuppressant therapy that was used as part of treatment. Relapse is more or less likely depending on factors such as the type of original cancer, its stage, and whether or not you were in remission at the time of the BMT. For those with acute diseases, such as leukemia, the odds that the disease will *not* return are highly favorable after a year or two has passed since the BMT.

It may take 3, 5, or more years of continued remission, though, before some physicians will consider a patient to be "cured." Because doctors and others in the medical community tend to talk more in terms of "unmaintained remissions" or "disease-free survival," you may not actually ever hear the word "cure" used. Some physicians don't feel comfortable using the word "cure" until you grow old and die of something else. Regardless of the semantics used, each year of cancer-free survival increases the odds that a permanent cure has been achieved.

After learning about all of the potential side effects and complications that can result during and after bone marrow transplantation, you may begin to wonder how anyone survives or goes on to live a rewarding life after this treatment. Be assured that many people do! A number of studies have examined the quality of life of long-term BMT survivors and support this fact. I am currently a participant in a 5-year quality-of-life research study being conducted at Johns Hopkins.

Because there is an ever-increasing number of persons undergoing and surviving BMT today, quality-of-life issues are moving to the forefront. Survival statistics alone don't describe how patients feel about their lives, how healthy they are, how they are able to function, or what side effects, if any, affect the quality of their lives following BMT. Therefore, a number of researchers have addressed this issue.

A study conducted by Schmidt and others[4] of 205 patients from City of Hope National Medical Center and 33 patients from Stanford University Hospital, who underwent allogeneic marrow transplants between 1976 and 1988, reported that "80% rated their 'quality of life' greater than 8 on a scale of 1–10." Karnofsky scores were "greater than 80% in 92% of the patients." (A Karnofsky score is a tool used by some medical researchers to assess a person's level of physical functioning. It is a scale that measures performance through a series of statements that rate physical ability along a continuum—anywhere from functioning independently at 100% in activities of daily living, to being disabled and requiring special help and care.) This study also reported that "82% of the patients were satisfied with their general appearance and 42% were gainfully employed."

A study by Chao and others[5] of 58 patients who underwent autologous BMTs at Stanford University Medical Center revealed that "88% of surviving adult patients reported an above-average to excellent quality of life 1 year following autologous BMT." It was also noted that approximately 78% of the patients were employed by the end of the first year after BMT. (Although some physicians and researchers view resuming employment and picking up where one left off in life as the gauge of a patient's return to physical and psychological health. Don't let this pressure you or make you feel badly about yourself or your recovery if you are not ready to re-adjust when it is expected.)

The *BMT Newsletter*, written and published by Susan Stewart, reported on "Long-Term BMT Survivors" in the January 1993 issue[6]. The twelve survivors that were interviewed all said they would make the same decision about choosing BMT. The newsletter noted that although they "identified continuing health effects from their transplant . . . most characterized the problems as minor when weighed against the benefits of transplant." The newsletter also reported on a 1990 survey conducted by Mel Haberman and Nigel Bush of the Fred Hutchinson Cancer Research Center. According to the newsletter, of the 125 BMT survivors (from 6 to 18½ years post-transplant) who participated, "77 percent of the long-term survivors surveyed by Haberman and Bush ranked their current physical health as good to excellent."

A study by Wingard and others[7] surveyed 135 patients from the Johns Hopkins Oncology Center who were between 6 and 149 months post-BMT. The study concluded: "Most subjects surviving marrow transplant reported good to excellent health and functional ability. [93% reported they could do normal activities with minor or no physical problems, Karnofsky scores were greater than or equal to 80%, and overall health was described as good to excellent by 67% of subjects.] Three-fourths were employed or enrolled in school. These outcomes are comparable to outcomes in survivors of cancer who received less intensive treatments." The study by Syrjala and others also reports favorably on patients' long-term employment following BMT, noting 68% had returned to full-time work 2 years after their transplants, and only 9% had not returned to full-time occupations by 4 years post-BMT.

A study by Belec[8], of 24 adults who were 1 to 3 years post-BMT, reports that "the majority of BMT recipients indicated that they enjoyed an acceptable quality of life." This was concluded because "approximately 92% of QLI (Quality of Life Index) scores were in the upper half of the possible range of scores." Lastly, in a study by Wolcott and others[9], of allogeneic marrow recipients treated at UCLA who were an average of 42 months post-transplant, it is noted that "of the 25 recipients who responded to the question about their current health, 4 (16%) rated it excellent, 13 (52%) rated it good, 7 (28%) rated it fair, and (only) 1 (4%) rated her health as poor."

Physical functioning and the perception of health can vary from patient to patient. The speed of recovery can vary as well. It is noteworthy that Syrjala and others reported that "recovery took longer than 1 year for approximately 40% (of the BMT survivors in their study)." Being aware of this may help patients who take longer than 1 year to recover feel less frustrated and disillusioned. It may be reassuring to their family members as well.

Although there are certainly some negative effects from BMT mentioned in each study cited, these studies invariably support the fact that the majority of surviving BMT recipients consider themselves to have a good quality of life following BMT. In spite of the fact that some of these studies surveyed a relatively small number of BMT survivors, the results for the most part are remarkably consistent.

Considering that patients treated with BMT have life-threatening illnesses prior to undergoing a transplant, and that this treatment itself is fraught with dramatic side effects and risks, these results are not only encouraging but may perhaps also be regarded as nothing short of miraculous. In light of all that patients go through to eventually become BMT survivors, the psychological and social implications from this experience must also be considered when evaluating the quality of life attained after bone marrow transplantation.

Psychological and Social Adjustment

There are bound to be some psychological aftereffects following BMT. Life-threatening illness itself brings with it a vast array of emotions, and undergoing BMT further adds to this because of its unique challenges. Although there can certainly be some lingering negative effects, many BMT survivors later identify a number of positive ways that this experience has affected the quality of their life.

Numerous factors influence your psychological and social wellbeing following BMT. In the research studies previously reviewed, physical health played a large role in determining how patients felt about their lives after BMT. Obviously, your physical condition influences your ability to live independently, hold down a job, pursue recreational activities, and other things that significantly affect your way of life.

In a study by Ferrell and others[10], being independent, healthy, normal, and able to work or achieve financial success were among the nine themes repeatedly identified by BMT survivors as important to their quality of life. Factors that can have an impact on your life after BMT include whether you have a job waiting for you after recovery, how understanding an employer is about your past health difficulties, and if you are able to resume your career.

The status of your relationships with both family and friends after BMT is also extremely important. These relationships may be viewed as being more valuable to you than they were in the past. Patients in Ferrell's study[11] identified "how often this value (of having family and relationships) was enhanced because of their experiences with BMT." Relationships can, however, undergo some profound changes both during and after treatment. They may be stronger, weaker, or just different somehow because of all you and those around you have been through. You may notice temporary or even permanent personality changes in you or in those around you. Some relationships may have even dissolved under the pressure of this lengthy and intense experience.

The responsibilities you held in your family before BMT and the roles you take on after BMT are also important to your emotional adjustment. Whether you are able to resume previous roles in your family, such as breadwinner or child-care provider, can change how you feel about yourself and your life. Previous responsibilities are often resumed gradually as you recover. These roles may undergo some permanent changes, however, sometimes by choice or necessity.

A change in priorities is also common after undergoing life-threatening illness and BMT. Life is often savored, appreciated, and enjoyed more. Belec's study of long-term survivors of bone marrow transplantation described it like this: "Recipients underwent a period of adjustment and adaption that was influenced by their experience with a life-threatening illness. During this period, a reappraisal or reassessment of life values occurred that positively affected their overall quality of life."

Ferrell and others[12] noted similar themes expressed by patients in their study, such as an "increased appreciation of life" and an increase in "spirituality." This study mentions that some BMT survivors feel increased religious faith, trust, and indebtedness to God after BMT. (It is my observation that some patients may also feel keenly indebted to those who supported them through the transplant. This sometimes results in exaggerated feelings of owing others or of guilt if the patient feels angry or disagrees with support persons (particularly the donor) in the future. Family members may also be overly protective of former BMT patients. Patients themselves may feel insecure after having been dependent on others for so long. In addition, it can be difficult to assume responsibility or feel comfortable socially right away.)

Ferrell's study went on to note that respondents mentioned that "a second chance [at life] was given" by BMT and that "transplants often resulted in a reevaluation of life priorities such that survivors were motivated to improve their situations." The second part of this study[13] noted that the appreciation for life was "followed by the need to now be productive." The researchers observed that, although achievement and fulfilling life's ambitions are positive goals, the BMT survivors felt "an urgent need to achieve after having been rescued from fatal illness."

Following recovery from BMT, patients can experience an intense need to make a difference in the world. You may feel that you have been saved for some higher purpose, or that you should now do something special with your life. There is no question that, for most patients, life certainly does feel more precious and worthwhile after BMT. The sheer joy of being alive, and the realization of how tenuous life is, can make you want to experience everything you've ever dreamed of as quickly as possible. For some this involves taking vacations, engaging in activities, or buying things they've always longed for. Some BMT survivors change careers or go back to school. The rush to get things done and experience all that life has to offer can sometimes, however, lead to physical exhaustion, financial indebtedness, and sleep difficulties.

Initially, some BMT survivors may even feel almost invincible because they survived such a serious disease and treatment. According to Belec's study several BMT survivors "expressed a sense of accomplishment at having survived BMT, and with the transplant behind them, they felt nothing could stand in their way." After being faced with the uncertainty of life, you may find that you live more for the present each day. Living only for today can make it more difficult, however, to make definite plans for the future. For some, even a few weeks from the present seems too far away to plan for.

Making or keeping commitments can also be more difficult if your health is not stable enough to predict whether you will be able to follow through with prearranged plans. Recognizing that life is short may cause you to be more giving or selfish with your time. Some BMT recipients feel a strong desire to help others who are battling cancer or who are about to undergo a BMT. Others would just as soon not talk about what they have been through and would rather put the BMT experience behind them.

Emotional distress is mentioned in most studies as a common problem following BMT. A study by Syrjala and others states that "patients and family members should be informed that emotional distress is normal, not only during the acute phase of transplantation, but also over the first year of recovery." This study further suggests that emotional concerns seem to become greater as physical concerns decrease. If patients and families understand that emotional fluctuations are normal and are experienced by many other patients as well, this may be less upsetting.

Studies have also been done to compare the emotional aftereffects experienced by BMT patients with those experienced by other patients to determine if BMT patients have more problems. A study by Lesko and others[14] found when comparing acute leukemia patients who received different types of treatments that "despite the additional strain and longer hospitalization associated with bone marrow transplantation, there was no difference found between BMT survivors and those treated with conventional chemotherapy alone in current psychological and social functioning." A study by Andrykowski and others[15] that compared BMT recipients to kidney (renal) transplant recipients found that "post-BMT QOL (quality of life) approximated that evidenced post-RT (renal transplant)." This is good news because it demonstrates that BMT survivors may experience similar outcomes as those who undergo other types of less dramatic treatments.

A number of research studies mention that the fear of a recurrence of the disease is another prevalent concern that can cause emotional distress for some BMT patients. This can continue to be a worry, not only during recovery but, in varying degrees, throughout life. That's not to say that most BMT survivors dwell on this fear, just that it is not unusual for this concern to surface occasionally. Sometimes, however, fear of relapse is less of a worry for BMT survivors than it is for those who have undergone more conventional forms of treatment. Ferrell and others[16] confirmed this by finding that a few of their respondents "felt that BMT had removed the fear of recurrence."

In the months and years that follow your BMT, it is not uncommon for disturbing memories of events that took place during your illness to surface occasionally. These flashbacks can conjure up strong, sometimes overwhelming, feelings of anxiety, fear, vulnerability, dependency, helplessness, isolation, frustration, loss, sadness, or depression. Intermittent periods of insomnia are not unusual. Reflecting on past experiences may keep you awake some nights. At other times, nothing specific may be wrong, but disquieting feelings may give rise to restlessness. Family members may experience these sleep disturbances as well.

When you experience minor illnesses in the future, even years after your BMT, you or your loved ones may again have flashbacks and have a recurrence of the strong emotional reactions that were experienced when you were seriously ill. Although this can be upsetting, and may even be perceived sometimes by others as overreactions or signs of poor coping, it is important to know that many patients and their loved ones have experienced similar feelings. Paying careful attention to your health and questioning even minor symptoms is certainly understandable considering all you have been through.

If you feel that post-BMT worries are interfering with your life or causing you continual stress, however, mention this to your doctor. Wolcott and others found that "15–20% of BMT recipient survivors report a degree of psychological distress that might benefit from specific psychological/psychiatric intervention." Individual counseling, family counseling, and attending support groups may all offer help in teaching you how to cope with these feelings. However, everyone has different needs and some patients find it more helpful not to talk about their past BMT experience. Emotional recovery, just like physical recovery, takes time. It is usually a gradual process that varies from patient to patient. Nevertheless, most patients and family members find that the frequency of traumatic memories and feelings does tend to decrease with the passage of time.

Just as those who have experienced the apparent randomness of casualties on the battlefield, BMT survivors may also experience "survivor's guilt" when seeing or hearing of others who die. Questioning why you survived and others did not is a normal reaction. This certainly doesn't negate feelings of being overjoyed and grateful because you have been cured, it's just that it can sometimes make you feel guilty and uncomfortable around other patients (and their families) who have not been as fortunate as you.

Another significant feeling expressed by a number of long-term BMT survivors is the feeling of being different from others, of not being "normal." In the study by Ferrell and others[17], it was noted that "respondents consistently referred to the lack of normalcy and the differences between themselves and those who have not experienced BMT." They mentioned that this was expressed not only by those with significant health problems but also for those with few chronic health problems. Belec reports that some of the long-term survivors in her study also addressed this issue. Belec said some stated that "they doubted that their lives ever would be the 'normal' that they knew before the transplant as their experiences had changed them." Although this theme is mentioned in many studies, don't assume that just because you may not feel the same as you did before your transplant that your "new normal" won't be as good or better than it was before your illness. There are bound to be some changes in your outlook and in how you feel about life.

Some of the emotional and physical post-transplant changes experienced by patients may seem particularly significant because most patients undergoing BMT are in the prime of their lives. A number of studies address this issue. Andrykowski and others[18] mention that the challenges of emotional readjustment for BMT patients are "certainly no different from those faced by cancer survivors in general. However, the impact of these challenges may be heightened because of the relative youth of BMT survivors. In contrast to many cancer survivors, BMT survivors must confront these challenges before or during the prime years of life. Thus, declines in physical, occupational, or financial status may have a more substantial and prolonged impact upon BMT survivors."

In light of the many adjustments BMT patients face throughout treatment and recovery, part 2 of the study by Ferrell and others[19] asked survivors, "What could physicians or nurses do to improve your quality of life?" The most common answer was to "be accessible." Some of the other responses were to "provide support groups," "provide additional coping strategies," "increase patient participation in decision making," and "reinforce current education (such as giving information that helps patients understand their symptoms, which symptoms are common, and what they may expect in the future)."

Belec pointed out that, in a study by Hengeveld, Houtmann, and Zwaan, recipients reported "feeling ill-prepared for the emotional and sexual problems experienced after discharge." This perhaps indicates areas where further help needs to be provided. It is not uncommon for patients and family members to express their wishes for additional support initially, as well as continuing support, from doctors and others in the medical community regarding what they have undergone and may still be experiencing. Some of the issues that warrant acknowledgment are the disruption and postponement of life plans and sadness at the inability to pursue plans that were previously important, but it can certainly help patients to know that most BMT survivors do eventually go on to enjoy many of the same things that others their age are experiencing.

Recovery from BMT unfolds over many months and years. Making the transition from patient to survivor often involves facing and overcoming some unpredictable and challenging obstacles. BMT is undeniably an experience that stays with patients and families for the rest of their lives. In spite of the physical and psychological difficulties that are encountered along the way, nearly all of the patients in the many studies previously cited, when asked, confirmed that making the decision to undergo BMT was the right choice. It is still the option they would have chosen knowing all they know now. BMT proved to be a life-saving treatment that enhanced their chances for long-term survival.

Again, besides the obvious positive physical outcome of being cancer free, most long-term BMT survivors also find that their BMT experience has improved the quality of their lives in many other less easily measured ways as well. Life is usually appreciated in a way that only those who have been faced with losing it can truly understand. Although life may never be quite the same as it was prior to BMT, it can be just as good or even better. Accepting what has happened in your life, no matter how hurtful or unfair it seems, and making up your mind to overcome past difficulties and move ahead, can be the first step in facing the future with renewed enjoyment, determination, and hope.

Dealing with Insurance and Financial Matters

No discussion on the topic of bone marrow transplantation would be complete without mentioning the issues of health insurance and the financial stresses that a treatment like BMT can generate. There is no getting around the fact that having a bone marrow transplant is very expensive. The cost is often estimated at around $150,000 or more. As some people are already painfully aware, insurance companies may refuse to provide coverage for this procedure. This is usually dependent on the patient's underlying disease and how well BMT is established as an accepted treatment. Even if coverage is provided, the massive quantity of paperwork, as well as the additional expenses of housing, transportation, and many others that accompany a treatment as technically involved and prolonged as BMT make this topic relevant to all patients and families.

Because most of us cannot afford to pay for a BMT without insurance coverage, this is the first hurdle that must be cleared—not only for peace of mind but for an easier entry into a BMT program. Those with certain types of cancer, such as leukemia or lymphoma, often have the easiest time obtaining coverage. BMT is accepted as a treatment for most kinds of leukemia when a perfectly matched, related donor transplant is proposed. On the other hand, those who have a less perfectly matched donor, an unrelated donor, or who have an autologous transplant, especially for certain solid-tumor malignancies, may have a much greater chance of being turned down for coverage by their insurance companies. Fortunately, more and more diseases are now being recognized by insurance companies as ones that necessitate treatment with a BMT. This is of little comfort, however, if your company is one that does not approve coverage.

If you receive an initial rejection from your insurance provider, there are a number of avenues you can pursue in an attempt to have the decision overturned. First, you must find out why you have been denied coverage in order to try to appeal and reverse the decision. Most often, it is because the procedure is deemed experimental. In this case it is necessary to enlist the aid of your physician, those at the transplant center, and/or evidence from previous studies that support the use of this procedure in treating your disease. If your insurance company considers BMT as "not medically necessary," have your physician submit additional medical information that supports why BMT *is* a necessary treatment for you. Obtain a second or even third physician's opinion that supports your doctor's decision, and include a review of current literature in the field that corroborates the use of BMT to treat your disease.

Find out who in your insurance company has decided against granting coverage and ask to speak with those who are higher up in the chain of command (supervisors, department heads, medical directors, etc.). At the first hint of insurance problems, take prompt and immediate action. Enlist help from the center where your proposed BMT is to take place, from your employer, and, if necessary, from an attorney to obtain approval. Don't give up or be intimidated easily. A little persistence and legal muscle may sometimes be all that are needed to turn the tide in your favor. The BMT Newsletter and the National BMT Link are two organizations that may be able to offer additional suggestions that can help you win coverage or refer you to an attorney who is skilled in dealing with this kind of case. Susan Stewart's book *Bone Marrow Transplants: A Book of Basics for Patients* has an excellent chapter on insurance and BMT, and Dr. Wendy Schlessel Harpham's book *Diagnosis: Cancer Your Guide through the First Few Months* has a short but informative section containing practical information on insurance, wills, and living wills that you may find helpful.

Even if you do not have trouble gaining approval for your BMT, there are many other insurance and financial issues you will need to deal with over the months, and often years, that follow your treatment. When the flood of bills, insurance forms, and explanations of benefits come rolling in, it can be overwhelming. Nevertheless, it is important to pay attention to these matters in a timely manner. Find a family member, friend, or professional service to take over or help out if you are too ill or are unable to handle this yourself. Some communications require a response, while others simply provide you with information, such as an assignment of benefits.

Try to promptly open and sort each bill or insurance statement as it is received. Keep *all* correspondence from the hospital, doctor, insurance company, and any other sources. Don't throw anything away until you are absolutely sure it will not be needed for future reference. It is often helpful to label manilla envelopes or folders with appropriate titles for the storage of such information. You may wish to label them by the institution or insurance company from which they came, or by the year or month in which they were incurred. Inpatient and outpatient bills can also be separated, as well as those that are paid and those that are outstanding. Use whatever system works best for you.

Make sure you review what your insurance policy covers and what deductibles you must pay. Question everything, unless you're sure it's not covered. If you do not know what your cumulative lifetime coverage amount is, find out. Whatever it is, it pays to conserve as many of your health care dollars for future use as possible. Once deductibles are met, don't be too hasty to pay fees that are decreed "not eligible" for coverage until thoroughly assessing them. When there are so many claims made over a short period of time, errors are bound to occur. *Carefully review each item on your billing invoice before paying anything.* I have been charged for procedures that were never performed, as well as for items that should have been covered and were inadvertently overlooked.

Also, pay special attention to outstanding differences you are charged for services considered above customary and usual fees for a particular medical item, drug, doctor's visit, or procedure. Charges for services in a metropolitan area or in a specialized field can sometimes cost more than those considered customary for your local area, therefore you may find that only a partial insurance payment will be made. For example, the fee for a doctor's visit at the BMT center may far exceed that of a doctor's visit in your area. Sometimes if you point out that specialized services are being provided, the charges may be fully covered. Sometimes a letter has to be written by a physician or billing source to explain why a procedure or service exceeds the cost that the insurance company permits. If all else fails, try to negotiate with the billing source to see if they will accept the fees that the insurance company deems as customary. Anytime you call or receive calls from the insurance company or from a billing office, record the date, time, and names of those you spoke with for future reference.

If you have an allogeneic transplant, donor costs are another area that can cause a great deal of confusion. These costs are the ultimate responsibility of the recipient and should be covered by his or her insurance provider. However, sometimes the recipient's policy dictates that they must first be submitted to the donor's insurance provider for rejection before they will be considered for payment. If the donor's insurance company decides to cover some of these costs it can really be confusing. This can further complicate the situation and make things difficult to straighten out. It can also make recipients feel uncomfortable or guilty, particularly if a donor is inconvenienced or bothered by requests for information from the hospital or insurance company.

If you end up owing legitimate uncovered expenses, which you undoubtedly will at some time or another, don't feel obligated to pay them off at one time if it creates undo financial hardship. Usually, you can set up a reasonable payment schedule with the billing source. You should take the time to call and explain your situation so a note can be made on your file. This can save you from getting upsetting letters in regard to collection. Don't let threatening words or letters intimidate you. If you make some monthly payment, no matter how small, it will show your intent to pay and, generally, no action will be taken against you.

Finally, before mailing in payments, carefully note the address where it is to be sent. Sometimes there can be subtle address differences on billing invoices that look virtually identical. If you write out one check and mail 2 or more invoices together, it can delay payment to the accounts that go to different departments or billing offices. What usually happens is that you will continue to get late notices requesting payment for the other accounts for months. This can be extremely irritating and frustrating, particularly when you know you have already paid them.

If your physician instructs you not to return to work within the first year post-transplant or if you have continuing health problems that keep you from returning to work, you may be eligible to apply for Social Security Disability benefits. The general criteria are that you must be considered disabled for a minimum time period of 1 year and that you must have contributed a sufficient number of years of work credit prior to your illness (usually 5 or more). If you meet these criteria, it may be well worth your time to contact a Social Security office for further information. The additional income, if you qualify, could help you meet the financial obligations remaining from your BMT, pay for new expenses incurred from continuing treatment, or offset daily living expenses until you get back on your feet. If you are approved to receive benefits, your children may be eligible to receive benefits as well (often one-half of what the parent receives) to aid in their support while you are disabled.

If you have private disability insurance or a work-related policy, it is important to notify the provider as soon as possible after your diagnosis to begin the benefit application process. Your policy dictates the circumstances that enable you to collect benefits and establishes when you are entitled to receive them. Your policy may specify a waiting period of 1 month, 3 months, or longer. If you are also eligible to receive Social Security Disability, you may be entitled to receive benefits from both concurrently, although the payment from the private source is often adjusted downward to reflect the additional income you are receiving from Social Security. Also, be aware that many disability insurance, life insurance, and other policies have a benefit that waives your premiums during the time that you are considered disabled. It is important to contact your agent to see if this applies in your case.

If you are ineligible for any kind of insurance coverage or benefits and are under great financial hardship, perhaps you will want to go public with your needs and set up a fund to accept donations from the surrounding community. Check with your local bank and attorney for the proper procedure to establish a special account. Fund raisers, donations from service and/or church groups, and financial aid from organizations (such as the American Cancer Society or the Leukemia Society of America) may provide additional support. Although it is often hard to accept financial help, or admit disability, these sources of financial assistance can be of great comfort to you and your family in getting through the months of recovery that lie ahead.

Once you have recovered, you may find that you encounter future problems with health and/or life insurance coverage or with job discrimination because of your history of cancer and BMT. A study of long-term BMT survivors by Belec found that an ". . . issue that presented itself was the employment difficulties experienced by recipients when attempting to re-enter society. Such difficulties also have been reported among other groups of BMT recipients and survivors of cancer." A study by Wingard and others found that "job discrimination and problems in obtaining insurance were reported by 23% and 39% [of the subjects], respectively." Although this study revealed that only a minority of patients were affected by these issues, it is nevertheless important to be aware of your rights in case it happens to you. The National Cancer Institute (NCI) has an excellent booklet entitled *Facing Forward—A Guide for Cancer Survivors*, which has two chapters on insurance and employment matters titled "Managing Insurance Issues" and "Earning a Living." A great many helpful suggestions are included; resources are given that help you better understand your rights under the law that prohibits discrimination, and additional avenues are recommended if you lose your health insurance or are turned down for coverage in the future.

Another source of information and support is the National Coalition for Cancer Survivorship (NCCS). This organization not only serves as a clearinghouse for information on a host of survivorship issues, but also serves as an advocate for the rights, interests, and study of cancer survivors. See the listing in the appendix to contact the NCCS for information or have your name added to their newsletter's mailing list.

References

1. Andrykowski, M.A., P.J. Henslee, and M.G. Farrall. "Physical and Psychological Functioning of Adult Survivors of Allogeneic Bone Marrow Transplantation." *Bone Marrow Transplantation* 4 (1989): 75–81.

2. Syrjala, K.L., M.K. Chapko, P.P. Vitaliano, C.Cummings, and K.M. Sullivan. "Recovery After Allogeneic Marrow Transplantation: Prospective Study of Predictors of Long-Term Physical and Psychological Functioning." *Bone Marrow Transplantation* 11 (1993): 319–327.

3. Wiley, F.M. and K.U. House. "Bone Marrow Transplant in Children." *Seminars in Oncology Nursing* 4 (1988): 31–40.

4. Schmidt, G.M., P.P. Fonbuena, N.J. Chao, B.A. Stallbaum, T.A. Barr, K.G. Blume, and S.J. Forman. "'Quality of Life' in Survivors of Allogeneic Bone Marrow Transplantation (BMT) for Malignant Disease." *Proceedings of the American Society of Clinical Oncology* (ASCO) 8 (1989): 311.

5. Chao, N.J., D.K. Tierney, J.R. Bloom, G.D. Long, T.A. Barr, B.A. Stallbaum, R.M. Wong, R.S. Negrin, S.J. Horning, and K.G. Blume. "Dynamic Assessment of Quality of Life after Autologous Bone Marrow Transplantation." *Blood* 80 (1992): 825–830.

6. Stewart, S.K. "Long-Term BMT Survivors." *BMT Newsletter,* no. 15 (January 1993).

7. Wingard, J.R., B.Curbow, F.Baker, and S.Piantadosi. "Health, Functional Status, and Employment of Adult Survivors of Bone Marrow Transplantation." *Annals of Internal Medicine* 114 (1991): 113–118.

8. Belec, R.H. "Quality of Life: Perceptions of Long-Term Survivors of Bone Marrow Transplantation." *Oncology Nursing Forum* 19 (1992): 31–37.

9. Wolcott, D.L., D.K. Wellisch, F.I. Fawzy, and J.Landsverk. "Adaption of Adult Bone Marrow Transplant Recipient Long-Term Survivors." *Transplantation* 41 (1986): 478–484.

10. Ferrell, B., M.Grant, G.M. Schmidt, M.Rhiner, C.Whitehead, P.Fonbuena, and S.J. Forman. "The Meaning of Quality of Life for Bone Marrow Transplant Survivors. Part 1: The Impact of Bone Marrow Transplant on Quality of Life." *Cancer Nursing* 15 (1992): 153–160.

11. Ferrell, B. and others. "The Meaning of . . . Part 1: The Impact . . . Life."

12. Ferrell, B. and others. "The Meaning of . . . Part 1: The Impact . . . Life."

13. Ferrell, B., M.Grant, G.M. Schmidt, M.Rhiner, C.Whitehead, P.Fonbuena, and S.J. Forman. "The Meaning of Quality of Life for Bone Marrow Transplant Survivors. Part 2: Improving Quality of Life for Bone Marrow Transplant Survivors." *Cancer Nursing* 15 (1992): 247–253.

14. Lesko, L.M., J.S. Ostroff, G.H. Mumma, D.E. Mashberg, and J.C. Holland. "Long-Term Psychological Adjustment of Acute Leukemia Survivors: Impact of Bone Marrow Transplantation Versus Conventional Chemotherapy." *Psychosomatic Medicine* 54 (1992): 30–47.

15. Andrykowski, M.A., E.M. Altmaier, R.L. Barnett, M.L. Otis, R.Gingrich, and P.J. Henslee-Downey. "The Quality of Life in Adult Survivors of Allogeneic Bone Marrow Transplantation: Correlates and Comparison with Matched Renal Transplant Recipients." *Transplantation* 50 (1990): 399–406.

16. Ferrell, B. and others, "The Meaning of . . . Part 2: Improving Quality . . . Survivors."

17. Ferrell, B. and others. "The Meaning of . . . Part 1: The Impact . . . Life."

18. Andrykowski, M.A. and others. "Physical and Psychological . . . Transplantation."

19. Ferrell, B. and others. "The Meaning of . . . Part 2: Improving Quality . . . Survivors."

Afterword

· · · · · · · · · · · · · ·

Nearly 5 years after my BMT, I am still free of leukemia. My bone marrow aspirations continue to show that my marrow consists of 100% healthy donor cells. My prognosis remains excellent. In spite of what I have been through, I am extraordinarily pleased with my life. I have been blessed with a wonderful family and caring friends. I remain positive by focusing on the wealth of personal growth and insight this experience has brought to my life. I choose to concentrate on what I have been given in life, not on what has been taken away.

I will always question, however, what caused me to develop leukemia in the first place. Of course, I look back and wish my illness had never happened. Yet, I love the person I am today, and I know I would not be this same person had I not been faced with the trials of a life-threatening illness. I also would never have met some of the marvelous people who have so enriched my life.

Although there have been changes, my life has taken on a comfortable new feeling of normalcy. Little day-to-day occurrences in life matter again, although minor aggravations do not bother me nearly as much as they once did. I appreciate my family and friends as never before and embrace new experiences with youthful enthusiasm. Although I've suffered, I've also been given a gift. The rare, beautiful gift of realizing just how precious life is. Each day is exciting and filled with endless possibilities. I know that it sounds like a cliché, but the blue sky really does look bluer, the grass does appear greener, and the sun seems to shine brighter than it ever did before.

Perhaps it's just that I take the time to notice these marvels more today than in the past.

Although many positive things have resulted from this experience, it's not to say that I don't have a few lingering physical and emotional aftereffects. Physically, I still have recurrent sinus and respiratory infections, skin sensitivities, and intermittent aches and pains in my joints. In the scheme of things, however, I feel these are rather minor side effects. Emotionally, some underlying fear, sadness, and pain still arise from time to time. It especially surfaces when I hear of others who weren't as lucky as I was and lost their battle with cancer. I realize that it could just as easily have been me and that at any time I could once again be thrust back into the fray. It comes out when I go to Johns Hopkins for my checkups and walk into the oncology center. I remember the difficult days of my own treatment and the sometimes heartrending experiences of the patients around me.

I do, however, credit the miraculous procedure of bone marrow transplantation for saving my life, and I applaud medical science for the advances that helped me to live. I will always be in awe of the early pioneers in the field of bone marrow transplantation, like Dr. George W. Santos and Dr. E. Donnall Thomas, who dared to dream that something like this could actually work and then went on to make it a reality. It will never cease to amaze me that someone's immune system can be successfully transplanted into another person's body.

Research is continuing, and advances are being made every day. Whether high-dose irradiation and/or chemotherapy followed by BMT will be the best treatment option for some cancer patients decades from now remains to be seen. Hopefully, newer treatments will be found or perfected that will only target cancer cells and spare normal body cells and organs from damage. If this proves to be routinely successful, it could very well eliminate the need for bone marrow transplantation and render it an obsolete treatment for cancer. At present, BMT continues to be the best or only hope, however, that some of us have for a second chance at life.

Along with many others, I have learned firsthand just how fragile and precarious our lives here on Earth can be. Therefore, it is important to live life to the fullest and to find joy in each day—you never know what tomorrow will bring. Don't wait until it's too late to tell your loved ones that you love them, and don't get so caught up in planning for the future or wallowing in the past that you forget to live today. If you feel the need to help others who have experienced cancer or who will be undergoing BMT, by all means search for the organizations, hospitals, and people that will support you in your efforts. No matter what contributions you make to society, find the niche in life that suits you best. What you make of the rest of your life is up to you!

It is a certainty that death and I will someday be face to face again. I pray that it will be when I'm old, after I've seen my son grow to become a man. I want to exit this world without regrets, with a peaceful grace that comes from having fulfilled my life's dreams. I hope that the information provided in this book has in some way helped you in your struggles if you're ill, or to more fully appreciate your health if you're not. For those who have never had to face their mortality, I hope it has given you some insight into what many of us who have been faced with the possibility of imminent death have experienced.

Writing this book was not an easy project. Researching and reliving each phase of the BMT process was at times emotionally difficult. I have tried, however, to portray the experience honestly and in a way that is as easily understandable as possible, considering the complexity of the subject. If this book educates the public and causes more people to become marrow donors or helps even one person feel less alone and more hopeful, then I have accomplished what I set out to do. I wish you all the best in whatever struggles you face and pray that you find all the peace and happiness in your life that I have eventually been so fortunate to find in mine.

Appendix

Resources

ORGANIZATIONS

Bone Marrow Transplant Information

The American Bone Marrow
Donor Registry

The Caitlin Raymond International
Registry of Bone Marrow
Donor Banks, Search
Coordinating Center
The University of Massachusetts
Medical Center
55 Lake Ave., N.
Worcester, Massachusetts 01655
(508) 756-6444
(800) 7-DONATE (for prospective
donors)
(800) 7-AMATCH (for patients)

Bone Marrow Family Support
Network
P.O. Box 845
Avon, Connecticut 06001
(203) 646-2836
(800) 826-9376

BMT Newsletter
1985 Spruce Ave.
Highland Park, Illinois 60035
(708) 831-1913

National BMT Link
29209 Northwestern Highway
#624
Southfield, Michigan 48034
(313) 932-8483

National Marrow Donor Program
(NMDP)
3433 Broadway Street NE
Minneapolis, Minnesota 55413
(800) 654-1247

International Bone Marrow
Transplant Registry (IBMTR)
Medical College of Wisconsin
P.O. Box 26509
Milwaukee, Wisconsin 53226
(414) 257-8325

Oncology Nursing Society
501 Holiday Dr.
Pittsburgh, Pennsylvania
15220-2749
(412) 921-7373

Cancer Information

American Cancer Society (ACS)
1599 Clifton Road NE
Atlanta, Georgia 30329
(800) ACS-2345

Leukemia Society of America (LSA)
600 Third Avenue
New York, NY 10016
(800) 955-4LSA

National Alliance of Breast Cancer
Organizations (NABCO)
Second Floor, 1180 Avenue of the
Americas
New York, NY 10036
(212) 719-0154

National Cancer Institute (NCI)
Cancer Information Service
9000 Rockville Pike
Bethesda, Maryland 20892
(800) 4-CANCER

National Coalition for Cancer
Survivorship (NCCS)
1010 Wayne Avenue
Fifth Floor
Silver Spring, Maryland 20910
(301) 585-2616

Oncology Nursing Society
BMT Special Interest Group
501 Holiday Dr.
Pittsburgh, Pennsylvania
   15220-2749
(412) 921-7373

PUBLICATIONS

BMT

Marget, Madeline. *Life's Blood*. New York: Simon & Schuster, 1992.
Stewart, Susan K. *Bone Marrow Transplants: A Book of Basics for Patients*.
   Highland Park, IL: BMT Newsletter, 1992.
Thompson, Francesca M., M.D. *Going for the Cure*. New York: St. Martin's
   Press, 1989.

Cancer

Bloch, Annette and Richard. *Fighting Cancer*. Kansas City: R.A. Bloch
   Cancer Foundation, 1985.
Cancer Manual. 8th ed. Boston: American Cancer Society, Massachusetts
   Division, Inc., 1990.
Coping: Living with Cancer. (magazine) 2019 North Carothers, Franklin,
   TN, 37064.
Dollinger, Malin, M.D., Ernest H. Rosenbaum, M.D., and Greg Cable.
   *Everyone's Guide to Cancer Therapy: How Cancer Is Diagnosed, Treated,
   and Managed Day to Day*. Kansas City: Andrews & McMeel, 1991.
Gaes, Jason. *My Book for Kids with Cansur*. Aberdeen, SD: Melius
   & Peterson, 1987.
Gravelle, Karen and Bertram A. John. *Teenagers Face to Face with Cancer*.
   New York: Julian Messner, Division of Simon & Schuster, 1986.
Harpham, Wendy Schlessel, M.D. *Diagnosis: Cancer Your Guide Through
   the First Few Months*. New York: W.W. Norton & Company, Inc., 1992.
Hirshaut, Yashar, M.D., FACP and Peter I. Pressman, M.D., FACS. *Breast
   Cancer: The Complete Guide*. New York: Bantam Books, 1992.
Mullan, Fitzhugh, M.D. *Vital Signs: A Young Doctor's Struggle with Cancer*.
   New York: Farrar, Straus and Giroux, 1983.
Noyes, Diane Doan and Peggy Mellody, R.N. *Beauty & Cancer: Looking and
   Feeling Your Best*. 2nd ed. Dallas: Taylor Publishing Company, 1992.

MEDICATION INFORMATION

Griffith, H. Winter, M.D. *Complete Guide to Prescription & Non-Prescription
   Drugs*. New York: The Putnam Berkley Group, Inc., 1993.
Long, James W., M.D. *The Essential Guide to Prescription Drugs*. New York:
   Harper Collins Publishers, Inc., 1993.
The PDR Family Guide to Prescription Drugs. Montvale, NJ: Medical
   Economics Data, Inc., 1993.

MEDICAL DICTIONARIES

Rothenberg, Mikel A., M.D. and Charles F. Chapman. *Barron's Medical Guide: Dictionary of Medical Terms*. New York: Barron's, 1989.

Thomas, Clayton L., M.D., MPH., ed. *Taber's Cyclopedic Medical Dictionary*. 17th ed. Philadelphia: F.A. Davis Company, 1993.

HOUSING AND TRANSPORTATION INFORMATION

Housing

Hope Lodge
c/o American Cancer Society
(800) ACS-2345*

Ronald McDonald House
Business office address:
500 North Michigan Avenue
Suite 200
Chicago, Illinois 60611
(708) 575-3429*

*or contact the social services department
at your prospective BMT center

Transportation

Corporate Angel Network, Inc.
Westchester County Airport
Building One
White Plains, New York 10604
(914) 328-1313

Glossary

A

Acute: having a rapid onset with severe symptoms and a short course.

Agranulocytes: one of the two main categories of white blood cells; named for the lack of granules (grainlike particles) in their cells; monocytes and lymphocytes are the two types of agranulocytes.

Alkaline phosphatase: an enzyme found primarily in the bones and liver. Elevations generally indicate disease in one or both of these areas.

Alkylating agents: a class of anticancer drugs that interferes with a cell's ability to divide by combining with its genetic material.

Allogeneic bone marrow transplant: a transplant that uses bone marrow obtained from a donor who is not genetically identical to the recipient; the donor and recipient are, however, usually a very close HLA match.

Alopecia: hair loss.

Anemia: a low red blood cell count.

Antibiotic: a medication that kills or inhibits the growth of bacteria.

Antibody: a protein made by the body's immune system in response to a specific foreign substance (called an antigen); if the same antigen invades the body again, certain white blood cells "remember" it and produce antibodies to destroy it.

Anticoagulants: agents that prevent or delay blood clotting.

Anticonvulsants: medications given to prevent or treat seizures.

Antiemetic: a medication given to prevent or stop vomiting.

Antigen: a substance that causes the immune system to produce antibodies.

Aplasia: when used in reference to bone marrow, means deficient or arrested blood cell production. A patient is generally considered to be aplastic (in a state of aplasia) when their neutrophil blood count is less than 500/cu. mm.

Asites: excessive fluid accumulation in the abdomen.

Autologous bone marrow transplant: a transplant in which the patient serves as his or her own bone marrow donor.

B

Bacteria: single-celled plantlike microorganisms. Some species are capable of invading body cells and producing disease.

Basophil: a type of white blood cell. Basophils are believed to be involved in allergic reactions and are sometimes found in increased numbers in association with tissue that is chronically inflamed or is in the process of healing.

B cell: a type of white blood cell that is involved in the production of antibodies; also called a B lymphocyte.

Benign: noncancerous.

Biopsy: the removal of tissue for microscopic examination.

Blast cell: a primitive, immature cell.

BMT: abbreviation for bone marrow transplant.

Bone marrow: a soft, jellylike/spongy substance found inside the cavities of bones that functions to produce blood cells.

Bone marrow aspiration: a procedure in which bone marrow is removed from the center of a bone for microscopic study. Most often removed from the iliac bones located above the buttocks.

Bone marrow harvest: the removal of a portion of bone marrow for use in a bone marrow transplant.

Bone marrow transplant (BMT): a procedure in which bone marrow is infused intravenously into a patient after he or she is treated with high-dose chemotherapy and/or total body irradiation.

Bone scan: a diagnostic medical test in which pictures are taken of the bones by a scanning machine after the injection of a radioactive substance into a vein.

Bronchiolitis obliterans: a serious lower airway disease caused by the inflammation and destruction of the small branches of bronchial tubes that lead to the lungs; can be a complication of graft-versus-host disease.

C

Cancer: a group of diseases characterized by abnormal cell growth and reproduction.

Carcinoma: a cancer that develops in the tissues that cover or line body organs.

Cardiac: concerning or involving the heart.

Cardiomyopathy: heart-muscle disease.

Cataract: a clouding over of the lens of the eye. Can be a late complication in bone marrow transplant patients who receive total body irradiation and/or steroid therapy; sometimes corrected surgically.

Catheter: a flexible tube inserted into a part of the body for the injection or removal of fluids.

CBC: abbreviation for complete blood count—a group of blood tests used to evaluate the type and quantity of blood cells present in the bloodstream.

Cells: the structural units that make up all living tissue.

Central nervous system (CNS): consists of the brain and spinal cord. Functions as the control center for the entire system of nerves located throughout our bodies. "Messages" must be sent back and forth through the central nervous system in order for sensations to be perceived, interpreted, and acted on.

Central venous catheter (CVC): a flexible tube that is surgically inserted into a large vein above the heart; sometimes referred to as a "central line."

Chemotherapy: treatment with one or more anticancer drugs.

Chromosomes: microscopic, rod-shaped structures, located in the center of the cells, which contain our genetic material.

Chronic: continuing for a long time, characterized by slow progression or little change.

CMV: abbreviation for cytomegalovirus.

CNS: abbreviation for central nervous system.

Colony-stimulating factors (CSFs): proteins that stimulate the growth and reproduction of certain kinds of blood cells in the bone marrow; CSFs are a category of growth factors.

Conditioning regimen: another name for preparative regimen.

Contracture: a permanent shortening of a muscle, joint, or the skin; can be a complication of graft-versus-host disease.

Corticosteroids: a group of drugs used to decrease inflammation and suppress the immune system. Used to treat and prevent graft-versus-host disease in BMT patients; commonly called "steroids."

Creatinine: a by-product of energy metabolism that is cleared from the body by the kidneys. Elevated levels of creatinine indicate impaired kidney function; normal blood levels are between 0.7 and 1.4 (mg/ml).

CSF: abbreviation for colony-stimulating factor. Can also be used as an abbreviation for cerebrospinal fluid, the clear, colorless fluid found within the brain and spinal canal.

CT scan: a diagnostic medical test that uses X rays to obtain cross-sectional views of body tissues; a contrast dye may be injected into a vein prior to the procedure; also called a "CAT" scan.

CVC: abbreviation for central venous catheter.

Cyclophosphamide: generic name for the drug known more commonly by the brand name Cytoxan.

Cystitis: inflammation of the bladder, usually caused by a urinary tract infection.

Cytomegalovirus (CMV): a type of herpes virus that can cause infection.

D

Diuretics: drugs used to increase urination.

DNA (deoxyribonucleic acid): a complex chemical compound that carries genetic information.

Dyspnea: shortness of breath.

E

Edema: swelling caused by the accumulation of fluid in body tissues.

EKG: an electrocardiogram—a test that records the electrical impulses of the heart.

Electrolytes: mineral substances found in our bodily fluids and tissues, such as potassium, sodium, and chloride; electrolyes are routinely measured as a part of patient assessment and care.

Emesis: vomit, vomiting.

Endocrine glands: glands in the body that secrete hormones, such as the pituitary, thyroid, adrenals, thymus, ovaries, and testes. Radiation and chemotherapy treatment can cause the endocrine glands to malfunction.

Engraftment: the process in which transplanted bone marrow migrates from the bloodstream to the bones and begins to produce blood cells.

Enzymes: protein substances produced by living cells that chemically react with other substances.

Eosinophil: a type of white blood cell; believed to combat certain parasitic infections and the allergens that cause allergies.

Erythrocytes: red blood cells.

Estrogen: the female sex hormone produced by the ovaries.

Ewing's sarcoma: a bone cancer primarily affecting children and young adults.

F

Fungus: a type of plantlike microorganism; some species are capable of causing infection in humans.

G

Gastric: concerning or involving the stomach.

Gastritis: inflammation of the stomach. Symptoms may include stomach pain, nausea, and vomiting. Gastritis can be caused by infection or by chemotherapy and radiation treatments.

Gastrointestinal (GI): concerning or involving the stomach and intestines.

G-CSF: abbreviation for granulocyte colony-stimulating factor; a type of protein that specifically stimulates the growth and reproduction of a type of granulocyte (neutrophils).

Gene: a unit of DNA, occupying a designated place on a chromosome, that is responsible for a specific inherited characteristic.

GI: abbreviation for gastrointestinal.

GM-CSF: abbreviation for granulocyte-macrophage colony-stimulating factor; a type of protein that stimulates the growth and reproduction of many different kinds of blood cells.

Graft failure: a complication following bone marrow transplantation in which marrow cells do not grow or are inadequate in number.

Graft rejection: a complication following bone marrow transplantation in which donor cells are rejected by immune cells of the recipient. For a patient with marrow cancer, this usually results in a relapse.

Graft-versus-host disease (GVHD): a condition that sometimes occurs after an allogeneic bone marrow transplant and in which immune cells in the transplanted (grafted) marrow launch an attack on body tissues of the recipient (host) because they are "recognized" as foreign.

Granulocytes: one of the two main categories of white blood cells. Named for granules (grainlike particles) that are present in their cells. Neutrophils, eosinophils, and basophils are the three types of granulocytes.

Groshong catheter: a type of central venous catheter. Groshong is the brand name.

Growth factors: substances that stimulate the growth of cells.

GVHD: abbreviation for graft-versus-host disease.

H

Hematocrit: the percentage of red blood cells in a given volume of blood; normally around 40–54 (%/100 ml) in men, 37–47 in women, and 31–43 in children.

Hematologist: a physician who specializes in the study, diagnosis, and treatment of blood disorders.

Hematology: the study of the blood.

Hemoglobin: the iron-containing pigment in red blood cells that carries oxygen from the lungs to body tissues; normally around 14–18 (g/100 ml) in men, 12–16 in women, and 11–16 in children.

Hemorrhagic cystitis: inflammation and ulceration of the bladder, generally causing pain and bleeding. A potential side effect from certain anticancer drugs, such as cyclophosphamide (Cytoxan) and ifosphamide.

Hepatic: concerning or involving the liver.

Hepatitis: inflammation of the liver.

Herpes simplex infection: a viral infection causing painful blisters on the skin or mucous membranes, commonly called "cold sores" or "fever blisters" when occurring around the mouth.

Herpes zoster infection: a viral infection caused by the varicella zoster virus that affects nerves. Produces painful skin eruptions along the affected nerves; commonly called "shingles."

Hickman catheter: a type of central venous catheter; Hickman is the brand name.

HLA: abbreviation for human leukocyte antigen.

Hodgkin's disease (HD): a cancer that originates in the lymphatic system, characterized by the presence of giant cells called Reed-Sternberg cells. It tends to spread in an orderly fashion from one lymph node to the next; also called Hodgkin's lymphoma.

Hormones: substances produced and released from endocrine glands or organs. They circulate in the blood and control other body cells by stimulating or inhibiting their activity or growth.

Human leukocyte antigen (HLA): a substance located on the surface of white blood cells that plays an important role in our body's immune response to foreign substances. These antigens are used to determine the suitability of a match between an organ donor and a recipient.

Hyperalimentation: intravenous solution that provides nutrition to patients who are unable to eat or cannot properly absorb nutrients from food; also called total parental nutrition (TPN) or hyperal.

I

Iliac bones: the large bones located in the pelvis: hip bones.

I.M.: abbreviation for intramuscular.

Immune system: the body's defense mechanisms that fight infection and foreign substances; consists primarily of white blood cells and antibodies.

Immunosuppression: a state in which the body has a decreased ability to prevent and fight infection.

Immunosuppressants: drugs that alter the body's immune system to prevent it from reacting against foreign substances.

Infertility: the inability to conceive or produce a child. It is a common side effect from some types of anticancer therapy; may be a temporary condition, not to be confused with sterility.

Infusion: the administration of fluids and/or medications through a vein into the bloodstream.

Interstitial pneumonitis (IP): a severe form of pneumonia within lung tissues; a complication that can sometimes occur in bone marrow transplant patients, most often caused by the cytomegalovirus (CMV).

Intramuscular (I.M.): within or into a muscle; a route used to administer medications by injection into a muscle.

Intrathecal: within or into the spinal canal; a route used to administer chemotherapy to the central nervous system.

Intravenous (I.V.): within or into a vein; a route used to administer fluids and medications directly into the bloodstream.

IP: abbreviation for interstitial pneumonitis.

Irradiation: therapeutic application of radiation to a patient or substance; radiation therapy.

I.V.: abbreviation for intravenous.

J

Jaundice: a condition in which body tissues take on a yellowish hue because of excessive accumulation of bile pigments in the blood, most often noticed in the skin and whites of the eyes. A symptom of liver disease or blocked bile ducts.

L

Laminar air flow: an air flow and filtration system that filters particles from the air and blows air along parallel lines at a uniform speed; sometimes used in bone marrow transplant units to help prevent infection in patients.

Late complication: when pertaining to bone marrow transplant patients, meaning a complication that occurs more than 100 days after the transplant took place.

Leukemia: a cancer that originates in the blood-forming cells of the body.

Leukocytes: white blood cells.

Liver function studies: a group of blood tests used to evaluate how well the liver is working.

Lumbar puncture: a procedure in which a needle is inserted into the spinal canal to remove a sample of cerebrospinal fluid for examination; also called a spinal tap.

Lymph: a clear, colorless fluid formed in the spaces between body tissues; it is gathered by way of lymph vessels and circulated in the lymphatic system before reentering the blood stream; differs from blood in that it does not contain red blood cells.

Lymph nodes: small, round structures of the lymphatic system that filter lymph of foreign matter. They produce lymphocytes and monocytes; those most easily felt are located in the neck, underarms, and groin.

Lymphatic system: a system of the body made up of lymph fluid, lymph vessels, lymph nodes, the tonsils, the thymus gland, and the spleen. It is a circulatory system in which lymph fluid is collected and drained from body tissues, filtered of foreign matter, and returned to the bloodstream; it plays an important role in the immune system.

Lymphocyte: a type of white blood cell that regulates the production of antibodies and destroys foreign substances in the body.

Lymphoma: a cancer that originates in the lymphatic system.

M

Macrophage: a type of white blood cell that has the ability to ingest and destroy invading organisms.

Malabsorption: a condition in which nutrients are not properly absorbed from the intestines.

Malignant: cancerous.

Metastasis, Metastasize, Metastatic: terms pertaining to the spread of cancer cells from the site of origin to other areas of the body.

Mixed lymphocyte culture (MLC): a lab test in which recipient and donor lymphocytes are mixed and cultured to determine if they react against one another.

MLC: abbreviation for mixed lymphocyte culture.

Monoclonal antibodies: highly specific antibodies that react against a specific antigen. They can be manufactured in a laboratory and used to "purge" bone marrow of certain cells before it is given to the recipient of a bone marrow transplant.

Monocyte: a type of white blood cell that serves as the body's second line of defense against invading foreign organisms.

MRI: an abbreviation for magnetic resonance imaging, a diagnostic medical test that creates detailed pictures of body tissues using a magnetic field and radio waves, instead of X rays.

Mucositis: inflammation of the mucous membranes (the layers of tissue that line body openings that are exposed to air); can produce discomfort, pain, ulcers, and/or excessive mucus production.

Multiple myeloma: a cancer that originates in the plasma cells of the bone marrow.

Myelocytes: cells in the bone marrow that mature into granulocytes.

Myelogenous: a term that means "originating in marrow."

Myelodysplastic syndrome (MDS): a group of cancers that originate in the stem cells of the bone marrow; characterized by the abnormal production of a wide variety of different types of blood cells (such as granulocytes, platelets, and erythrocytes); chromosomal abnormalities in the cancer cells are common.

N

Nadir: low point; used to refer to the lowest level blood cell counts will reach after anticancer treatment.

Neuroblastoma: a cancer that originates along the nerves that run from the base of the skull down into the pelvis; usually occurs in infants and children.

Neurologic, neurological: concerning or involving nerves.

Neutrophil: a type of white blood cell; the most numerous and important kind of granulocyte in terms of protecting us from bacterial infections. Also called a "poly."

Non-Hodgkin's lymphoma (NHL): a type of cancer that originates in the lymphatic system; the name given to a wide variety of lymphomas, excluding Hodgkin's disease.

N.P.O.: abbreviation meaning nothing by mouth (no eating or drinking); commonly ordered the evening prior to surgical procedures.

O

Oncologist: a physician who specializes in the study, diagnosis, and treatment of cancer.

Oncology: the study of cancer.

P

Palliative: treatment given to relieve disease symptoms; not intended or expected to produce a cure.

Peripheral edema: swelling in the arms or legs due to fluid accumulation in body tissues.

Peripheral neuropathy: numbness or tingling in the extremities, most often in fingers or toes, caused by damage to nerves; a side effect that can occur from certain types of anticancer treatment.

Peripheral stem call harvest: the removal of stem cells from the bloodstream for later use in a bone marrow transplant; stem cells are removed in a procedure that involves withdrawing blood through an intravenous catheter and circulating it through a cell-separating machine.

Peripheral stem cells: pluripotent stem cells found circulating in the bloodstream.

Petechiae: small, red pinpoint areas of bleeding on the skin; usually caused by a low platelet blood count.

Plasma: thin, colorless or faint yellow fluid that serves as the medium in which blood cells circulate; the liquid part of the blood and lymph.

Plasma cells: cells of the immune system that produce antibodies; plasma cells are made when B lymphocytes come into contact with particular foreign antigens.

Platelets: blood cells that help control bleeding by causing the blood to clot; also called thrombocytes.

Pluripotent stem cells: primitive blood cells, found primarily in the bone marrow, which are capable of reproducing and differentiating to make all varieties of mature blood cells. They are also found circulating in the bloodstream, but in much smaller quantities. Pluripotent stem cells are usually referred to as "stem cells."

Pneumonia: inflammation of the lungs, generally caused by infectious organisms.

Pneumonitis: medical word for pneumonia.

P.O.: abbreviation meaning to take by mouth, to swallow.

Polys: another name for neutrophils.

Preparative regimen: anticancer treatment given prior to a bone marrow transplant, consisting of total body irradiation (TBI) and/or high-dose chemotherapy; also called conditioning regimen.

Protective isolation: the physical isolation of a patient in a protective environment to try and prevent infection. It often requires visitors and medical personnel to wear gowns, gloves, and facemasks; also called reverse isolation.

Protocol: a plan of medical treatment to combat disease.

Pruritus: severe itching.

Pulmonary: concerning or involving the lungs.

Pulmonary fibrosis: the formation of scar tissue in the lungs; can be a complication from anticancer treatment.

Purging: the removal of certain cells from the bone marrow before it is given to the recipient of a bone marrow transplant. Usually refers to the removal of cancer cells in an autologous transplant or T cells in an allogeneic transplant.

R

Radiation therapy: anticancer treatment in which high-energy radiation is administered to the body; also called radiotherapy.

RBC: abbreviation for red blood cell.

Red blood cells: cells in the blood that carry oxygen from the lungs to body tissues and then transport carbon dioxide back to the lungs to be exhaled; also called erythrocytes.

Relapse: the recurrence of disease after it appeared to have been eradicated.

Remission: a complete or partial disappearance of cancer cells and symptoms; not necessarily a cure.

Renal: concerning or involving the kidneys.

Retinoblastoma: a cancer originating in the retina, the thin layer of tissue lining the back of the eyeball. Occurs primarily in very young children and is sometimes an inherited disease.

Rhabdomyosarcoma: a cancer that originates in muscle tissue; the most common soft-tissue sarcoma found in children.

S

Sarcoma: a cancer that originates in bones, muscles, or tissues that support and connect other tissues.

Secondary malignancy: a cancer that develops after treatment for another kind of cancer; can be a late complication caused by previous radiation therapy or chemotherapy; also called secondary cancers or secondary tumors.

Seizure: a sudden, involuntary attack of muscle contractions and relaxations; also called a convulsion or a "fit."

SGOT: abbreviation for serum glutamic oxaloacetic transaminase, an enzyme present in highly active body tissues, such as the heart and liver. Elevations indicate tissue disease or damage.

SGPT: abbreviation for serum glutamic pyruvic transaminase, an enzyme found in high concentrations in the liver. An elevated SGPT is a more specific indicator of liver disease or damage than is an elevated SGOT.

Shingles: see herpes zoster infection.

Solid tumors: carcinomas and sarcomas.

Splenomegaly: enlargement of the spleen.

Sputum: a relatively clear mucous substance expelled by coughing or clearing the throat. When discolored or produced in excessive quantity usually indicates the presence of infection or disease.

Staging: medical testing done to evaluate how far a cancer has spread in the body.

Stem cells: see *pluripotent stem cells.*

Sterility: the inability to conceive or produce a child; usually used to denote a permanent condition.

Steroids: see *corticosteroids.*

Stomatitis: inflammation and soreness of the mouth.

Syngeneic bone marrow transplant: a transplant that uses bone marrow obtained from an identical twin.

System: when used in reference to the body, means an organized grouping of related structures that work together to perform certain bodily functions.

T

TBI: abbreviation for total body irradiation.

T cell: a type of white blood cell that attacks substances in the body which are recognized as not belonging to "the self"; also called "killer T cells" and T lymphocytes.

T-cell depletion: removal of a portion of the T cells from donor bone marrow before it is given to the recipient. The aim is to prevent or lessen the symptoms of graft-versus-host disease.

Thrombocytes: platelets.

tissues: a group of similar cells that work together to perform a particular body function.

Total body irradiation (TBI): the exposure of the entire body to gamma radiation; used as an anticancer and bone marrow destroying treatment prior to bone marrow transplantation; usually given in a number of separate doses over the course of several days.

Total parental nutrition (TPN): intravenous solution that provides all of a patient's nutritional requirements; also called hyperalimentation.

TPN: abbreviation for total parental nutrition.

Transplant: to transfer or implant tissue from one part of the body to another or from one person to another.

Tumor: a mass, swelling, or enlargement; a new growth of tissue. May be benign or malignant.

Tumor burden: the quantity of abnormal cells that are present in the body.

U

Ulcer: an open sore.

Ultrasound: a diagnostic medical test that uses sound waves to create pictures of body tissues.

V

Varicella zoster virus (VZV): the virus that causes shingles and chicken pox.

Venocclusive disease (VOD): a potential complication after high-dose chemotherapy and/or radiation treatment in which the blood vessels of the liver become blocked and damaged.

Virus: an extremely small microorganism that is dependent on other organisms to live and reproduce; certain species are capable of causing infection in humans.

VOD: abbreviation for venocclusive disease.

W

WBC: abbreviation for white blood cell.

White blood cells: cells in the blood that fight infection; also called leukocytes.

Wilms' tumor: a relatively rare childhood cancer that originates in the kidneys.

Index

·········

About the Author

Marianne L. Shaffer, a former BMT patient, is a registered nurse who holds a Bachelor's Degree in Psychology. She has completed specialized training in providing one-to-one support for cancer patients and their families through the CanSurmount program of The American Cancer Society and has experience serving on the Cancer Response System hotline (for the state of Pennsylvania), a nationwide information service established by The American Cancer Society. Throughout her career, she has worked in patient education, both before and after her own illness, which served as the compelling motivation to write this book. She resides in Dillsburg, Pennsylvania, with her husband, Tim, and their son, Kevin. *Bone Marrow Transplants: A Guide for Cancer Patients and Their Families* is her first book.